Thieme

Yamamoto New Scalp Acupuncture

Principles and Practice

Richard A. Feely, DO, FAAO, FCA, FAAMA

Adjunct Associate Professor
Department of Osteopathic Manipulative Medicine
Chicago College of Osteopathic Medicine
Midwestern University
Downer's Grove, IL, USA

2nd edition

90 illustrations

Thieme
Stuttgart · New York

Library of Congress Cataloging-in-Publication Data
is available from the publisher.

Important note: Medicine is an ever-changing science undergoing continual development. Research and clinical experience are continually expanding our knowledge, in particular our knowledge of proper treatment and drug therapy. Insofar as this book mentions any dosage or application, readers may rest assured that the authors, editors, and publishers have made every effort to ensure that such references are in accordance with **the state of knowledge at the time of production of the book.**
Nevertheless, this does not involve, imply, or express any guarantee or responsibility on the part of the publishers in respect to any dosage instructions and forms of applications stated in the book. **Every user is requested to examine carefully** the manufacturers' leaflets accompanying each drug and to check, if necessary in consultation with a physician or specialist, whether the dosage schedules mentioned therein or the contraindications stated by the manufacturers differ from the statements made in the present book. Such examination is particularly important with drugs that are either rarely used or have been newly released on the market. Every dosage schedule or every form of application used is entirely at the user's own risk and responsibility. The authors and publishers request every user to report to the publishers any discrepancies or inaccuracies noticed. If errors in this work are found after publication, errata will be posted at www.thieme.com on the product description page.

Illustrators: Christy L. Kelley, Chicago, IL, USA, and
Anthony M. Pazos, Mesa, AZ, USA

Rüdigerstrasse 14, 70469 Stuttgart, Germany
http://www.thieme.de
Thieme New York, 333 Seventh Avenue,
New York, NY 10001, USA
http://www.thieme.com

Cover design: Thieme Publishing Group
Typesetting by Sommer Druck, Feuchtwangen, Germany
Printed in India by Gopsons Papers Ltd, Noida

ISBN 978-3-13-141832-6 1 2 3 4 5 6

To Carol, Brad, and Ashley

Foreword

Dr. Feely has not only been to numerous YNSA seminars, including those at my hospital, but has also arranged for me to give seminars several times in Chicago. Now after he has studied the subject of YNSA thoroughly, he has formulated it well into TCM thoughts and teachings in ways that I had never even thought of when developing my method and working with it for many years.

The Chinese proverbs that are included support the YNSA teachings. I think many TCM followers will understand the system better now that it has been presented in their frame of reference. Whatever the thought or formulation, the main aim of YNSA is to help the patient. This, I am sure, is also Dr. Feely's main object.

I sincerely wish Dr. Feely great success with his book as well as with his work.

Toshikatsu Yamamoto, MD, PhD

Preface to the Second Edition

This edition, like the first edition, provides a connection for those knowledgeable in other forums of acupuncture, TCM, Eight Principles, Five Phases, and French Energetics school of acupuncture, to relate to, and add YNSA to their therapeutic armamentarium.

The previous edition of this book was very well received by the profession, with many more people in the English-speaking world taking up YNSA as a therapeutic treatment method for millions of suffering patients. Fortunately for the human race, the science of medicine and the knowledge acquired of the human body continue to expand exponentially. We now know much more about the biochemistry of the brain and the neurotransmitters that are associated in the metabolic cascade of pain and the perception of pain.

Some of the protocols have been refined and have become more specific with some new points. This new edition goes into greater detail regarding the electromagnetic field and physiology of the human body and its potential.

Currently, most of the YNSA research continues to be carried out in Europe and Asia. It is hoped that controlled scientific experimentation, verifying or disproving YNSA diagnostic, treatment protocols, and point location will be undertaken in US institutions.

In this edition, you will find:

- New points
- Improved graphics
- New case reports
- A new chapter on energetics.

We have included the best parts of the first edition, particularly the DVD, and the clinical aid diagnostic/treatment card, as well as all the protocols that have been proven effective.

I trust that you will find this work easy to read, providing excellent instruction, inspiration, and guidance in diagnosing and treating your suffering patients.

Richard A. Feely

Preface to the First Edition

When one has been on a journey for two decades, it is not uncommon to wonder how it all started. For me, it began in Kirksville, Missouri, where as an undergraduate I became exposed to osteopathic medicine, a holistic philosophical approach to medicine, and discovered that osteopathy was also my personal philosophy. Osteopathy, philosophically, states that the body is a unit where structure and function are reciprocally interrelated, and that the body has homeostatic mechanisms that a wise physician uses and relies upon in promoting health. This form of medicine, which looks for and promotes health and not disease, made the most sense to me. Therefore, I became a Doctor of Osteopathy (D.O.).

After completing a pre-doctoral fellowship in osteopathic theory and methods, specifically manipulation, and post-doctoral training, I embarked on the practice of osteopathy. One day I had metatarsalgia and went to a colleague, a well-trained osteopathic physician specializing in manipulation, who proceeded to suggest that he treat this pain with acupuncture. He placed a few needles in my foot, leg, and arm, and the pain abated. Intrigued with this response, I decided to pursue the acquisition of knowledge to determine the flow of energy (*qi*) using acupuncture as a means of balancing and harmonizing the body, similar to my treatment goal in utilizing osteopathic manipulative techniques.

As a cranial osteopath, I was trained in diagnosis and treatment from a Western perspective—anatomy, physiology, and pathology—but with the added knowledge, skill, and ability of palpating the primary respiratory mechanism/craniosacral mechanism, thus, perceiving the life energy, as expressed in the neuromusculoskeletal system. Cranial osteopaths learn how to move the fascia, body fluids, ligaments, and *qi* with their hands through the restricted areas of the body, bringing life to diseased and dysfunctional tissues.

My interest peaked with that personal experience and I subsequently enrolled in the UCLA Medical Acupuncture Course for Physicians by Dr. Joseph Helms. I continued to participate in many other professional acupuncture educational activities. On one such occasion in Arizona, I met Toshikatsu Yamamoto, M.D., Ph.D., the founder of Yamamoto New Scalp Acupuncture (YNSA). With that one meeting, my life and my patients' lives have been changed, as we together experienced the pain-relieving, life-changing energy of a needle properly placed in the scalp.

Here is one of those life-changing stories. It was Wednesday afternoon as I walked into the middle treatment room of my downtown Chicago high-rise office to find my next patient, Mary, curled up in the fetal position with the lights off and her husband, Jim, quietly sitting in the chair next to her. Jim spoke up, "She's still having her headaches, migraines that she has had continuously for five years." After failing with two famous, world-class headache centers and many other doctors between Albuquerque and Chicago, Jim and Mary had come from New Mexico to see if I could help her with my unique combination of techniques. They were desperate for a miracle but discouraged and armed for further disappointment. After a complete history, physical, and osteopathic structural examination, I confirmed the diagnosis of recurrent classical migraines with concomitant muscle tension cephalgia along with somatic dysfunction of the head; the cervical, thoracic, and lumbar spine; the sacrum; and the pelvis. I recommended that we begin treatment with cranial osteopathic manipulation followed by YNSA. After her cranial osteopathic treatment, she stated she was 60% better. She had less pain and she was able to open her eyes with the lights on. I then placed six needles in her scalp as the Yamamoto neck diagnosis protocol indicated and she said, "I can see! I feel good! This is the first time in five years I don't have a headache! Whoa!"

In 1994, I traveled to Miyazaki, Japan, from Chicago to spend time with this unique man, Toshikatsu Yamamoto, M.D., Ph.D., whom I had met previously in Arizona at the national meeting of the American Academy of Medical Acupuncture. I was amazed at what I saw and learned. There I saw this slight, Japanese physician place four to five needles in the scalp of a hemiplegic patient and immediately the patient was able to move their paralyzed limb!

With such dramatic physical changes using only a few needles, I was intrigued, to say the least. At my next opportunity, I was to find myself in Japan at Dr. Yamamoto's hospital on the neurological wards. One after another, post-stroke (CVA) patients would get their usual four to eight needles in the scalp and they *all* would begin moving their paralyzed limbs. I couldn't—more accurately—*I would not believe* it because everyone was getting better right before my very eyes. It was too good to be true! Then Dr. Yamamoto placed his usual needles in the scalp of a 70-something-year-old, right hemiplegic lady and nothing happened—*THEN, that is when I believed* Dr. Yamamoto's technique, YNSA, was real and not magic, because in medicine nothing is always perfect. Unfortunately, in medicine some patients do not always respond, even when the physician does everything correctly. Like any other medical therapy, YNSA works well for many conditions but it is not a panacea.

This book is a compilation of both Dr. Toshikatsu Yamamoto's pioneering work and my latest diagnostic and treatment points as identified in over 10 years of YNSA practice. The reader will find new and a few different points than those listed in Dr. Yamamoto's 1998 book, *YNSA*. I have started and continued with Dr. Yamamoto's nomenclature. I then expanded and refined the YNSA numbering system to provide a common language for use with current US medical documentation and CMS insurance requirements for correct E/M coding and acupuncture procedures documentation (see **Table 7–1**, page 90).

Since YNSA is a science of the 21st century and is neither widely known nor practiced, very few research papers and rigid scientific studies have been completed on it. Most of the evidence on the effectiveness of YNSA is from case reports and small studies by individual physicians in Japan, Europe, and the United States. In Dr. Yamamoto's book, *YNSA*, he lists 30 case reports of the effects of YNSA on circulation, quadriplegia, aphasia, tinnitus, facial paralysis, herniated lumbar discs, knee pain, tension headaches, cervical spondylitis, shoulder pain, compression fracture, cerebellar hemorrhage, post-CVA hemiplegia, Raynaud's disease, herpes zoster, cerebral concussion, and cerebral contusion with tetraplegia. He also lists the results of the use of YNSA Basic points for pain relief and hemiplegia. He reports that YNSA consistently provided pain relief to patients, yielding 72–85% marked improvement with Basic points A, B, C, D, and E (n = 253, 1855, 2593, 25 844, 130 respectively). He also reported that of the 483 hemiplegic patients, 55% had marked improvement if treated within the first 30 days following CVA. If treated within the first 6 months following CVA, 43% had marked improvement. If treated between 6 and 12 months following CVA, 35%. And if treated over 1 year later, 14%. Stating it in the negative, of the 483 hemiplegic cases that were treated over 1 year later, no improvement was seen in 28%; and for those treated between 6 months to 1 year, no improvement was seen in 25%.[1]

In conclusion, most of the YNSA points in this book were discovered by Dr. Yamamoto and a few by me. These points were identified based upon Dr. Yamamoto's YNSA microsystem theory, TCM, and the Five Phases principles combined with individual trial and error. Currently, YNSA is ready for high-quality scientific scrutiny by the acupuncture world with controlled research trials to verify or disprove the diagnosis and treatment methods presented in this book. There is a need to have controlled scientific experimentation, verifying or disproving point location. Research is also needed to prove the value and the correctness/usefulness of terminology for each of the points presented in this book.

This book was designed to aid the student/practitioner in learning and reviewing his/her YNSA point location and to help improve the understanding of the YNSA diagnostic and treatment protocols. To practice YNSA, one has to develop a microsystem intellectual framework and proper psychomotor skills in mastery of the YNSA diagnostic and treatment systems. This is best taught one-on-one, with a student treating a suffering patient under the guidance of a wise and experienced teacher. In such situations, results, often dramatic, can readily be seen. Perfect practice makes for accurate diagnosis and truly effective treatment.

As you, the physician and/or acupuncturist begin your study of YNSA, may these words, thoughts, and charts provide you with knowledge, perfected in wisdom, to enable you to deliver superior healthcare to your suffering patients.

Richard A. Feely

References

1. Yamamoto T, Yamamoto H. Yamamoto New Scalp Acupuncture (YNSA). Tokyo, Japan: Axel Springer Japan Publishing, Inc.; 1998 : 191, 193.

Acknowledgments

The appreciation for the individuals who have helped me in my journey regarding YNSA starts with Toshikatsu Yamamoto and his energetic wife, Helen. His discovery and tenacity to continue this new work since first presented in 1973 is a testimony to him and all those physicians who allow their patients to teach them the truth of physiology in clinical practice.

I would like to thank Angelika Findgott, Birgitta Brandenburg, and Anne Lamparte for their editorial encouragement and professionalism.

For helping me to provide quality clinical care to the patients developing the YNSA protocols, I wish to thank my medical assistants, Kathy Moran and Debbie Barton.

I wish to give special thanks to Rocio Galvan for her hard work in helping me transcribe and Laura Cauldwell for proofreading this text.

Finally, I thank my lovely wife Carol for her constant support.

Table of Contents

1 Introduction to Yamamoto New Scalp Acupuncture (YNSA)

"To live in harmony with yin *and* yang *means life: to act contrary to them means death."*[1]

"Aspire to the principle, behave with virtue, abide by benevolence and immerse yourself in the arts." – *Chinese Proverb*

What is YNSA. A complete acupuncture microsystem of the scalp utilizing Basic (anatomical) and Ypsilon (channel) points to affect the human body through the bioelectric and biochemical systems, enabling the patient to move toward balance and harmony, which is health.

History of YNSA. Discovered by Toshikatsu Yamamoto, MD, PhD, Miyazaki, Japan, in 1973 and currently practiced in Japan, Europe, North America, Brazil, and Australia.

YNSA success. Thousands of patients have received pain relief and restored health utilizing YNSA for such infirmities as stroke, herniated discs, chronic fatigue, fibromyalgia, and migraine headaches, to name a few.

While treating patients in his hospital and clinic, Toshikatsu Yamamoto, MD, PhD, of Miyazaki, Japan, discovered and developed a new system of scalp acupuncture, Yamamoto New Scalp Acupuncture (YNSA). He first presented this system of scalp acupuncture at Ryodoraku Congress in Osaka, Japan, in 1973. Dr. Yamamoto then developed the YNSA system of neck and abdominal diagnostic procedures coupled with scalp, chest, and pubis microacupuncture treatment. He did this while caring for patients with acute and chronic neurological conditions at Yamamoto Hospital in Nichinan, Japan.

Overview

YNSA is a microsystem of acupuncture. Dr. Ralph Alan Dale of Miami, Florida, introduced the term *microacupuncture* at the 1974 Third World Symposium on Acupuncture and Chinese Medicine. Dr. Dale defined microacupuncture as the expression of the entire body's *qi* in each major anatomical region.[2] Microacupuncture systems have been identified by Dale on the ear, foot, hand, scalp, face, nose, iris, teeth, tongue, wrist, abdomen, back, and every long bone of the body. Each region is a functional microcosm of the traditional energies of the whole body. Every part of the body contains the representation of an energetic microorganism through microacupoints and microchannels that reiterate the topology of the body.[3]

The Microsystems

An acupuncture microsystem is defined as a single part of the human body that, when accessed, can directly influence the entire body's *qi*, blood, and moisture—from the organ to the cellular level—resulting in changes of physiology and symptomatology.[4] Every microsystem manifests neurological reflexes connected to parts of the body that are remote from the anatomical location of that particular microsystem. These reflexes can be both diagnostic and therapeutic. They can be activated by acupuncture needles, massage, moxibustion, heat, electrical stimulation, and magnets. Locations of distant tender points are not random but are related to the neurological reflex pattern that is centrally mediated. The microsystem reflex map of the body represents the anatomical arrangement of the whole body. *Somatotope* means representative body area or map. The somatotope of YNSA is oriented in an upright pattern and its representation is ipsilateral, which means same side; that is, if the right shoulder hurts, the YNSA acupoint will be most likely on the right side of the scalp. Furthermore, there are bidirectional connections in the microsystem point when pathology is in a specific organ or body part, which is indicated by changes in the skin conductivity; thus, stimulating that microsystem point can produce changes in the corresponding parts of the body. Cutaneous stimulation triggers nervous system messages to the spinal cord and brain, activating bioenergetic changes, biochemical exchanges, and alterations in the electrical firing of neuronal reflexes.

All microacupuncture systems interact with the macroacupuncture systems; the 12 regular, paired channels, the two single midline channels, and the eight extraordinary vessels. Therefore, the treatment of one system will produce changes in the body's functional patterns as diagnosed by other systems. Treatment of the overall macrosystem affects the functioning of the microsystems.[3] The bioelectrical and biochemical effects of placing a needle on the scalp will be discussed in Chapter 2. One of the current theories of how this microsystem of acupuncture may work is explained in the Fractal Field Model of the structure of the organism, which will be explained later in Chapter 2.[4] YNSA is a somatotopic representative microsystem. The entire body is anatomically and functionally represented on the scalp in an upright manner (**Fig. 1–1**).

YNSA utilizes two types of needling categories: (1) Basic, which correspond with anatomical locations and (2) Ypsilon, which correspond to the 12 paired acupuncture channels. The Basic points correspond to the axial and appendicular neuromusculoskeletal structures. The Ypsilon points are representative of the 12 channels of body acupuncture. The 12 channels are shown in **Table 1–1**.

To determine the necessity for these Ypsilon points, Dr. Yamamoto developed a specialized palpatory neck diagnostic procedure called YNSA

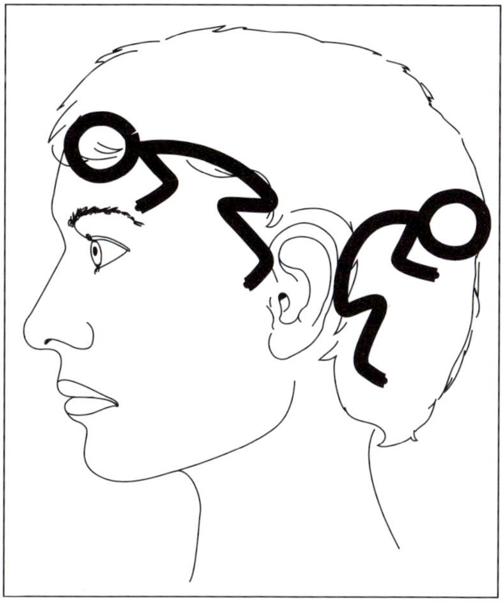

Figure 1–1 *Yin/yang* somatotope.

Table 1–1 The 12 channels

Organ Point Channel	Standard Abbreviation
Lung	LU
Large intestine	LI
Stomach	ST
Spleen	SP
Heart	HT
Small intestine	SI
Urinary bladder	BL
Kidney	KI
Pericardium	PC
Triple burner	TB
Gall bladder	GB
Liver	LR

neck diagnosis, which will be discussed in Chapter 5.

To date, YNSA's greatest use is in the treatment of pain and neuromusculoskeletal dysfunction and disease. Clinically, YNSA is amenable to both hospital and outpatient settings. Starting with the patient's history and presenting complaint(s), adding a standard medical physical examination combined with the YNSA neck diagnosis procedure, a skilled practitioner is provided with all the information needed to render a YNSA diagnosis and deliver a high quality YNSA treatment. Utilizing YNSA neck diagnosis to determine which Basic and Ypsilon points need treatment, one is able to be very specific and effective in achieving a balance of *qi*, blood, and moisture, thereby harmonizing the body's bioelectric system with just a few needles.

Traditional Chinese Medicine (TCM) acupuncture is the body acupuncture system consisting of over 365 acupuncture points (acupoints) strung together in 14 meridians or channels. TCM is the macrosystem of acupuncture. It is classical, channel-based acupuncture, where all acupoints are defined by a channel and correlate with specific acupoint functions, effects, and spirit; some of these functions include entry/exit, *luo* connection, *xi* cleft, and *yuan* source. The YNSA microsystem honors and recognizes the important functions, effects, and spirit of the TCM channels and their points. YNSA Ypsilon points encapsulate all those points' actions within the TCM channel into just one acupoint on the scalp. There are many macroacupuncture or TCM acupoints on the scalp, including the gall bladder (GB), bladder (BL), triple burner (TB), governing vessel (DU), and stomach (ST). With rare exceptions, YNSA points are not the same acupoints at all. This YNSA system is not a macro or body acupuncture system.

YNSA is an acupuncture microsystem that is different, yet similar, in some aspects from the other well-known microsystems: Chinese and French Auricular, Korean Hand, and Chinese Scalp Acupuncture. The Chinese and French Auricular systems are limited to the ear for diagnosis and treatment. The Chinese and French auricular systems are derived from TCM. "The theoretical origins of auricular therapy derive in the first instance from classical descriptions of the pathways of the channels (meridians). Of the twelve primary channels (meridians), the six yang channels skirt portions of the ear either directly or through a branch channel and the six yin channels have no direct connections, but are nevertheless indirectly linked through their inner and outer relationships with the yang channel."[5] "More than 200 acupuncture sites were charted on the auricle by Chinese medical workers."[3] Auricular points are named for their corresponding anatomical part, or effect[3]; these range from purely anatomical to functional to psychological states of being.[2] With the use of a device measuring electrical resistance on the auricle of the ear, research in Europe, America, and Asia has found the auricle to be diagnostic and therapeutic in treating a variety of diseases.[3]

Auricular acupuncture (ear acupuncture) has both functional and anatomical points. It also has acupoints that relate to the progression of illness in the four phases, which, when identified during the corresponding phase of health (or illness), are amenable to effective treatment. Auricular diagnosis often uses an acupoint finder and treatment with electrical stimulation of the point. The late Paul Nogier, MD, of France, discovered and developed the three somatotopic phases of illness progression in ear acupuncture as described in his 1981 book, *De L'Auriculotherapie a L'Auriculomedicine*, which was translated in 1983 to *From Auriculotherapy to Auriculomedicine*. This work discusses the three phases, which he defines as ectoderm, mesoderm, and endoderm; he later added the fourth phase, neuromusculoskeletal, on the back of the pinna which largely relates to the neuromusculoskeletal system.[6] These four phases are related to, and correspond to, the progression of disease within the human body.

Auricular acupuncture is often done using an electronic detection device that can be both diagnostic and therapeutic. Using Dr. Nogier's phases and an electrical device, one is able to follow the progression of reflective changes in the disease state as it goes from affecting the superficial to internal organ, and from internal organ to deeply affecting the patient's mind and finally the spirit. Like Nogier's auricular acupuncture, YNSA has four phases of treatment.

- Phase 1 Ectoderm treated in Yin of YIN for Superficial (acute) illness/dysfunction
- Phase 2 Mesoderm treated in Yang of YIN for Organ dysfunction/disease
- Phase 3 Endoderm treated in Yin of YANG for Mind/cognate dysfunction/disease
- Phase 4 Neuromusculoskeletal treated in Yang of YANG for Spirit and severe disease

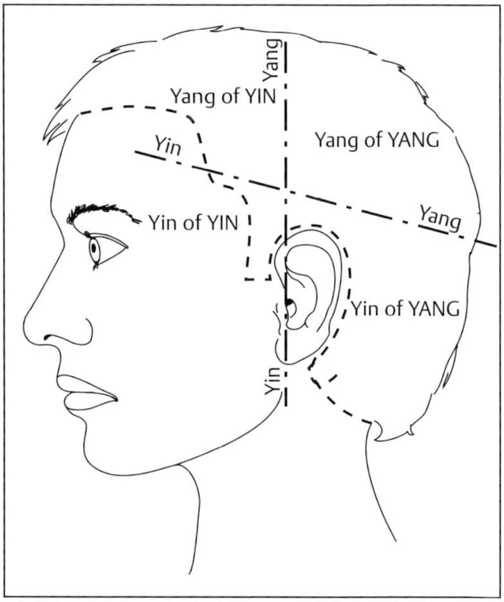

Figure 1–2 Lateral four quadrants.

The phases represent the progression of illness over time and the severity of disease. The French auricular four phases are similar to the four YNSA Ypsilon quadrants (Yin of YIN, Yang of YIN, Yin of YANG, and Yang of YANG), as illustrated in **Fig. 1–2**.

Korean hand acupuncture is a microsystem of the hand only. "As far back as the interclassic, it is suggested that certain diseases can be treated by stimulating the points on the side of the body opposite that of the disease."[7] "This principle of contralateral treatment is generally applied to hand acupuncture, the disease affecting the left side of the body is treated by inserting needles into the right hand and vice versa."[8] These points are named for their anatomical and functional relationships. YNSA is different; it treats points ipsilaterally on the scalp.

Although the traditional Chinese Scalp Acupuncture (CSA) is a microsystem of the scalp like YNSA, it uses a different somatotope than YNSA.[8] CSA has been shown to be particularly effective in treating strokes and cerebral vascular conditions similar to Dr. Yamamoto's reports regarding utilization of YNSA. While there are two scalp microsystems indicated by Dale in 1976, the principle system divides the temporal section of the scalp into three parts. A diagonal line is extended laterally from the top of the head to the area of the temporals above the ear. The lowest portion of this temporal line relates to the head. The middle area relates to the body, arms, and hands. The uppermost region relates to the legs and feet. This inverted body pattern represented on the scalp activates reflexes in the ipsilateral cerebral cortex to the contralateral side of the body.[9]

Today, there are five main sects of CSA. The first is Jiao's Head Acupuncture, which is based on scalp area zones that correspond to the functional location of the cerebral cortex. It is involved in more than 40, mainly cerebrogenic, diseases.

The second is Fang's Scalp Acupuncture, which is based on superimposing pictures of the spine and the human body in a prone position on the scalp. Its main indication is for cerebrogenic diseases and eye diseases.

The third is Tang's Head Acupuncture, which is based on the location of the function of the cerebral cortex in combination with the TCM theory of *zang fu* organs. The main locations for the acupuncture needles are the forehead and temporal regions of the scalp that are divided into two parts—the front (with the supine human body superimposed) and back (with the prone human body superimposed)—both of which are divided into forehead and face zones. There are zones of upper, middle, and lower *jiao*, etcetera. The main indications are wide and varied in addition to central nervous system diseases.

The fourth is Zhang's Treatment, which is based on the location of the acupuncture points in certain treatment zones. Manipulation of the acupuncture needle in the scalp is primarily the rotational method. The main indications are nervous and mental diseases only.

The fifth and last main sect of CSA is Zhu's Scalp Acupuncture, which is based on theories of *zang fu* organs and channels. The main indication is hemiplegia due to apoplexy. The secondary indication is to treat emergent and severe diseases of various clinical entities. The international standard plan for the acupoints of scalp acupuncture has four regions. The forehead region has four standard lines. The vertex region has five standard lines. The temporal region has two standard lines. Lastly, the occipital region has three standard lines. Zhu's Scalp Acupuncture, in America, is the more popular of the five sects.

CSA is concerned with more directly influencing the brain's motor centers by placing stimulating needles directly over these centers where there are motor and pre-motor cortexes. Finally, Drs. Dan Bensky and John O'Connor, in *Acupuncture: A Comprehensive Text,* sum up CSA nicely, saying "generally a principle site is selected which corresponds directly to the representative area on the cerebral cortex for a certain disease and a supplementary site may be added which is less directly related."[10]

Auricular and hand acupuncture are like YNSA in that they are true microsystems affecting the patient's entire body with organ, channel, and bodily function points, albeit needling a different body part to have an effect. YNSA is different from all other microsystems in that it has an additional unique palpatory diagnostic system, YNSA Neck Diagnosis, to determine which Ypsilon (channel) point is to be used. Although TCM (Eight Principles/Five Phases) body macroacupuncture systems use acupoints on distinct channel lines that are connected to and go through/around the head, YNSA does not; it has only one point per channel in each of the four quadrants. YNSA has a microsystem of Basic Points related to kinesic body parts or anatomical sites plus the Ypsilon Points, related to the 12 channels: lung (LU), large intestine (LI), stomach (ST), spleen (SP), heart (HT), small intestine (SI), bladder (BL), kidney (KI), pericardium (PC), triple burner (TB), gall bladder (GB), and liver (LR). The Basic points are usually found in the medial aspect of the scalp, whereas the Ypsilon points are found in the lateral temporal area of the scalp.

YNSA Diagnosis and Treatment

YNSA has two main systems for practical diagnosis and treatment: To diagnose, YNSA utilizes history and palpation. Palpation means YNSA Neck and/or Abdominal Diagnosis Systems and is used as the means to determine which Basic and/or Ypsilon points are tender and thus need acupuncture.

For treatment, YNSA places needles in scalp Basic points, which are anatomically related (**Figs. 1–3 and 1–4**), and/or Ypsilon points, which are channel related and representative of the 12 Primary (*zang fu*) channels (**Fig. 1–5**). Basic points are determined by history, YNSA Neck/Abdominal Diagnosis points, and direct Basic point scalp

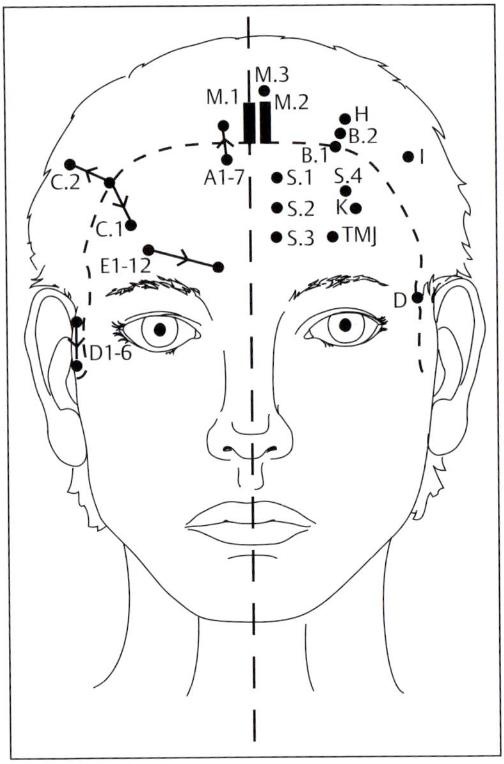

Figure 1–3 Anterior *yin* Basic points.

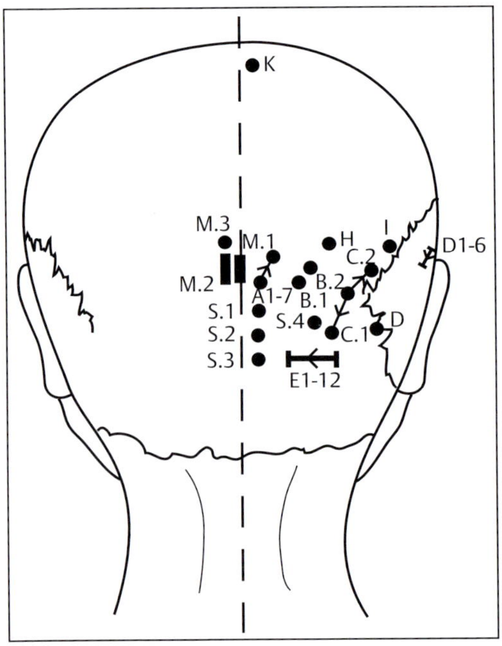

Figure 1–4 Posterior *yang* Basic points.

Table 1–2 Representative characteristics of *yin* and *yang* principle states

Yin	*Yang*
Female	Male
Soft	Hard
Lower	Upper
Moist	Dry
Dark	Light
Night	Day
Interior	Exterior
Cold	Hot
Blood	*Qi*/energy
Retiring	Active

palpation for tenderness with palpable subcutaneous tissue elevations in the scalp. Ypsilon points are primarily diagnosed by using YNSA Neck/Abdominal Diagnosis points followed by Ypsilon point palpation for tenderness and/or subcutaneous tissue elevation in the scalp. The entire length of each channel is encapsulated in the respective Ypsilon point.

These YNSA Ypsilon and Basic points are further divided into two principle states: YIN and YANG. The representative characteristics of each are given in **Table 1–2**.

YIN, by definition, is the ventral or anterior half of the body and/or lower part of the scalp. YANG, by definition, is the dorsal or posterior half of the body and/or upper part of the scalp. Each of the principle states is further divided into two subdivisions making up one of the four YNSA quadrants. YIN is further subdivided into Yin of YIN (**Fig. 1–6**) and Yang of YIN (**Fig. 1–7**). YANG is further subdivided into Yin of YANG (**Fig. 1–8**) and Yang of YANG (**Fig. 1–9**).

All Basic points are divided into Yin and Yang, which roughly represent the homunculus as depicted previously in **Figure 1–1** and now also in **Figure 1–10**. The Yin is in the inferior half of the scalp and the Yang is in the superior half of the scalp. Basic points are found in the frontal area and are called Yin, specifically Yin of YIN. Basic points found in the occipital area are called Yang,

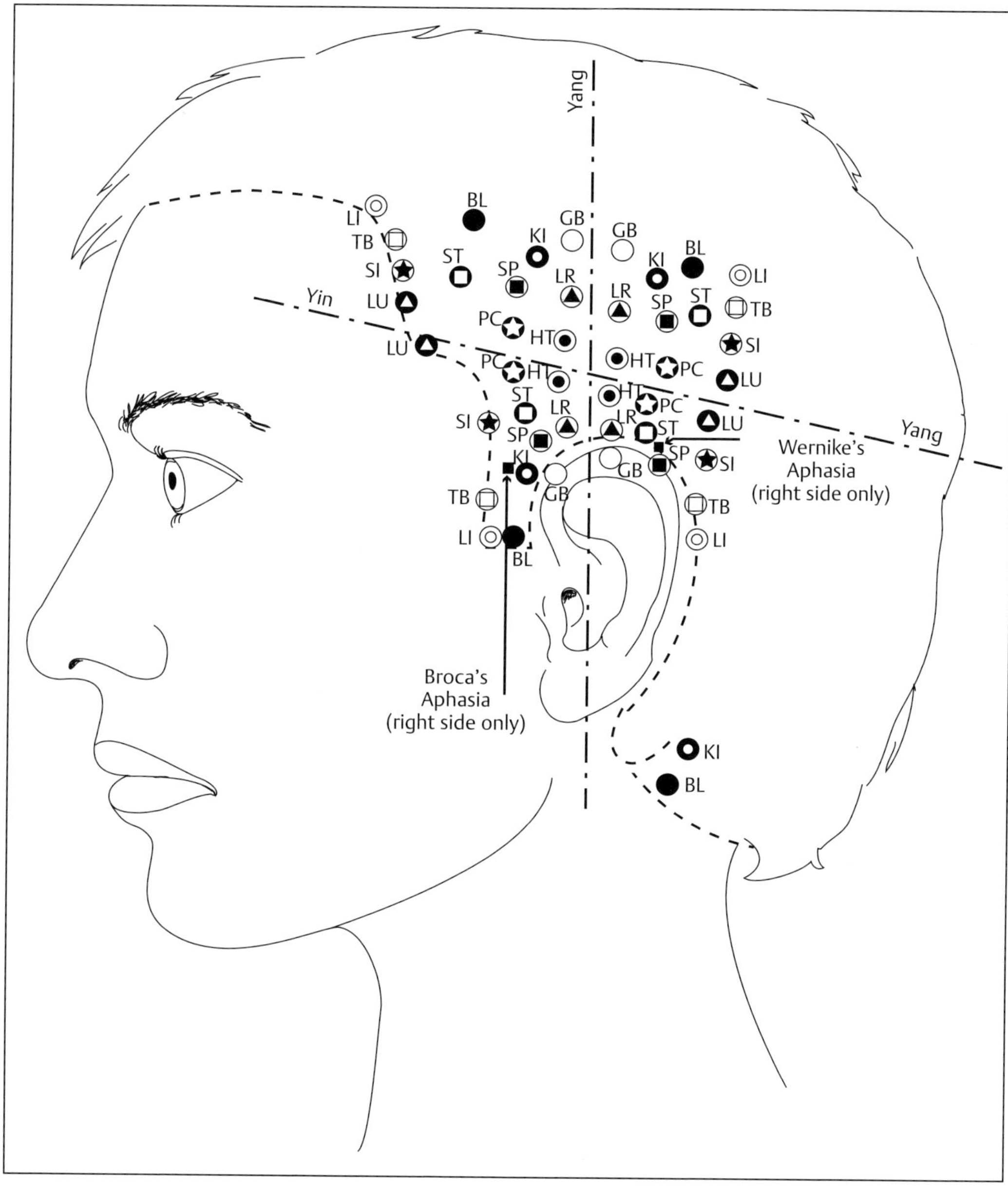

Figure 1–5 Lateral *yin/yang* Ypsilon points.

specifically Yin of YANG. The head is divided at Du-20 (*bai hui*), the anterior vertex of the scalp is Yang of YIN Basic points and posteriorly to Du-20 (*bai hui*), the vertex of the scalp is Yang of YANG basic point (**Fig. 1–11**).

Ypsilon points also have two principle states: Yin and Yang. Both are present on both the left and the right side of the head. Within the left and right side of YIN, there is Yin and Yang. Within the left and right side of YANG there is Yin and Yang. The result is four quadrants on the left and four quadrants on the right. These four quadrants of Ypsilon points are Yin of YIN, Yang of YIN, Yin of YANG, and Yang of YANG, either left or right, as seen previously in **Figure 1–2**. The location of the Ypsilon points in the four quadrants correlates

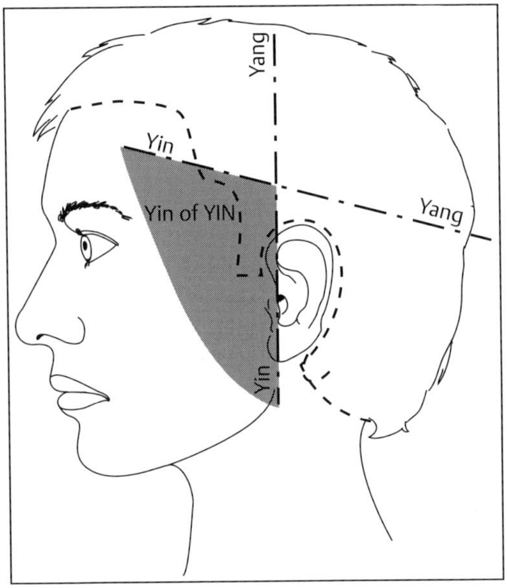

Figure 1–6 Lateral Yin of YIN quadrant.

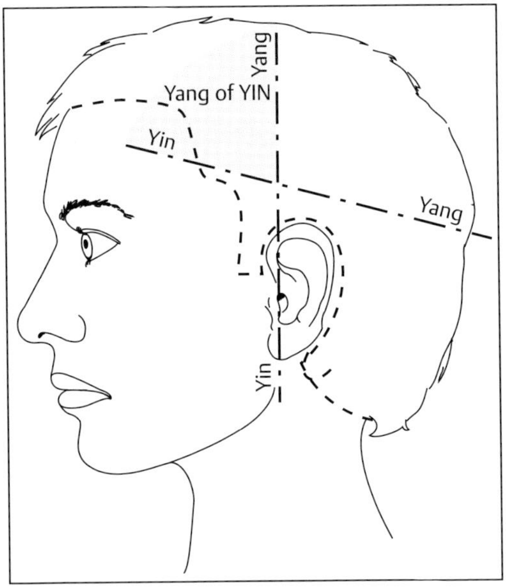

Figure 1–7 Lateral Yang of YIN quadrant.

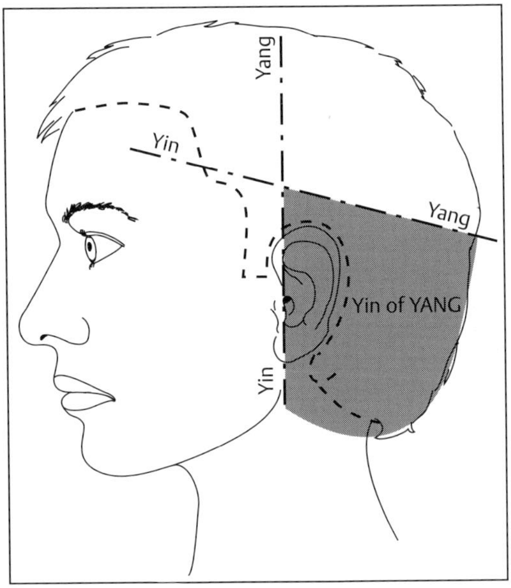

Figure 1–8 Lateral Yin of YANG quadrant.

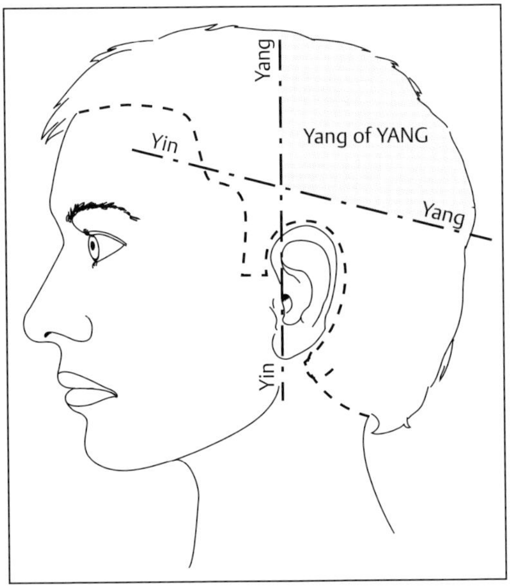

Figure 1–9 Lateral Yang of YANG quadrant.

with the four phases of health similar to Nogier's four phases in auricular acupuncture.

Two principle categories of YNSA points are:

- Basic points
- Ypsilon points

Two sides of Basic and Ypsilon points:

- Left
- Right

Two principle states of Basic and Ypsilon points:

- Yin
- Yang

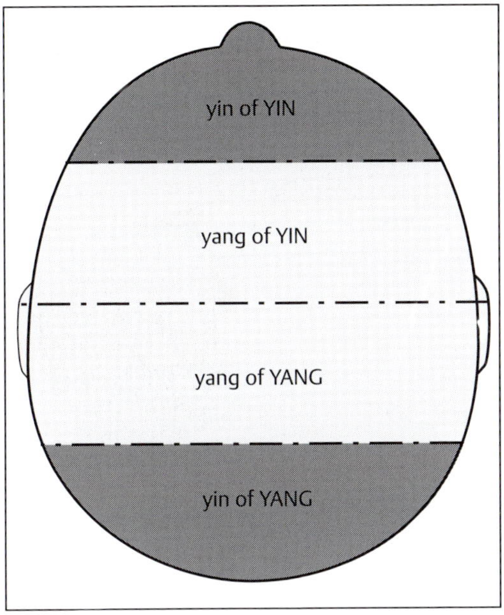

Figure 1–10 Crown somatotope YIN and YANG.

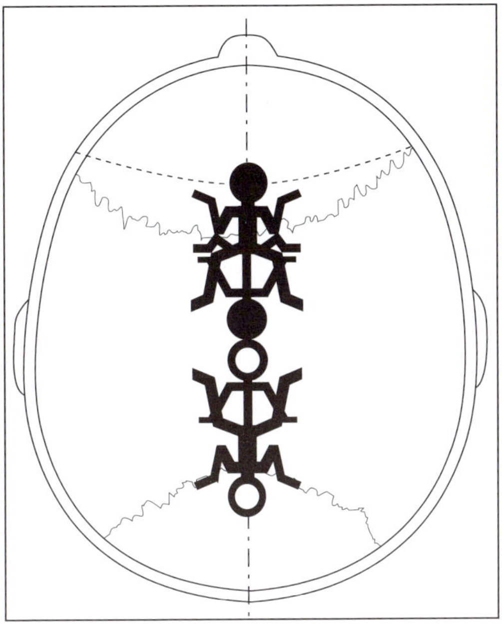

Figure 1–11 Crown of four quadrants.

Four quadrants of Basic and Ypsilon points:

- Yin of YIN
- Yang of YIN
- Yin of YANG
- Yang of YANG

In conclusion, YNSA's microsystem of acupuncture was originally developed focusing on the scalp. The Basic points cover regional body parts, including arm, leg, regions of the spine, cerebrum, cerebellum, and specialized points for sciatic, tinnitus, aphasia, and cranial nerves. The Ypsilon points directly relate to the 12 *zang fu* acupuncture channels, see **Table 1–1**, with *Ren*/conception vessel and *Du*/governing vessel not yet separately identified. The YNSA Neck and Abdominal Diagnostic System is used to identify which Ypsilon points require treatment based on palpatory tenderness and quadrant.

YNSA and Acupuncture Integration

YNSA provides both diagnostic and therapeutic acupuncture microsystems designed for relieving both somatic and visceral problems through the modulation of neurotransmitters, affecting pain, and ultimately by balancing the 12 *zang fu* acupuncture channels effecting pernicious influences, in addition to *qi*, blood, and moisture within the TCM paradigm.[11]

With the addition of Five Element/Five Phases and TCM knowledge, one is able to use the Ypsilon points more efficiently and effectively to harmonize and balance these 12 channels. Successful treatment can be clinically verified through the physiologic feedback loop as demonstrated by lack of tenderness in YNSA neck diagnosis points or normalized TCM (Eight Principle/Five Phase) pulse diagnoses after correct placement of YNSA needles. The pulse diagnostic system immediately indicates a more balanced pulse after proper needle placement. The YNSA Neck Diagnosis procedure improves immediately to no tenderness after correct needle placement. Thus, one is able to treat the patient in a complete, holistic, balanced, and harmonic way using YNSA.

It is the author's opinion that any microsystem cannot provide the same exact effect on the human body, mind, and spirit as the three main macrosystems, TCM, Five Element/Five Phases, and French Energetics. There is no YNSA point to represent the spirit of the acupoint, such as KI-24 (*ling xu*), "absence of spirit". There are no YNSA points to represent the function of the entry and exit points. There are no YNSA points that exactly represent triangular equilibration with progression. And finally, there are no YNSA points that are as effective for removing blocks as Five Phase treatments, such as Internal and External Dragons. After all, YNSA is a microsystem, a shorthand way to get the body's attention to change and become balanced, but it cannot compete with all the nuances of the macroacupuncture system's content of clinical effect, spiritual effect, and a single macroacupuncture point's specific physiological effect. However, the shorthand macroacupuncture system provides a quick, powerful effect with a few needles to balance and harmonize the body's system and uniquely affect the central nervous system.

With this elaborate YNSA microacupuncture system, using the knowledge of Five Phase acupuncture and TCM, a practitioner can easily focus the treatment approach to the patient in quite an elegant way, often with only a few well-placed YNSA needles. For example, a patient with asthma might have positive left Yin of YIN KI and LU by YNSA neck diagnosis points. To treat, the practitioner would simply needle these two left Yin of YIN YNSA Ypsilon points, KI and LU. Then, the practitioner would recheck the YNSA neck tenderness and/or Five Phase/TCM pulse diagnosis for verification of a successful treatment. With only two needles, the YNSA practitioner has affected *tai yin* (LU) and *shao yin* (KI), the mother and the son, the original *qi* and the source *qi*.

YNSA is most often used as a stand-alone treatment but may in certain circumstances be used as reinforcement to other moderate to light macroacupuncture treatment approaches. For example, in a case with pelvic pain, one may use YNSA Basic point C-2 for the pelvis and the *dai mo* extraordinary channel for treatment of pelvic pain. Another example, with the TCM diagnosis of deficient blood causing decreased memory in a 60-year-old, is using YNSA points M-2, HT, KI, and SP to tonify blood. In addition, one may add TCM macroacupuncture sea of blood points, ST-37, ST-39, and BL-11. YNSA also may be quite effectively used on the same day with other forms of treatment such as injections, medication, psychotherapy, physical therapy, and manipulation, which will be covered more in Chapters 10 and 13.

It is by placing all the needles in the correct Ypsilon quadrant, over the correct representative channels, that one can produce a beautiful, electromagnetic harmonic wave, thereby affecting the brain. This bioelectrical and biomechanical effect of the needle is transmitted through the fascia and mesodermally derived structures to the rest of the body. The end result is balanced *qi*, blood, and moisture flowing through all channels. This is done through proper placement of needles using the YNSA methodology, which effectively purges pernicious influences and enlivens the eight principles (e.g., strengthen heart, purge phlegm, and tonify moisture, which, in turn, restores joy and fluidity within the patient's physiology and psychology).

YNSA Utilization

This YNSA system is particularly good at helping treat pain, neurological conditions, and organ dysfunctions. YNSA may be used in a variety of medical, surgical, and pain conditions either as primary treatment or as secondary/complementary treatment. In all surgical and most medical cases, it will be complementary and not the primary treatment because many diseases and medical conditions have very effective Western medical treatment protocols. The best medical care requires a skilled physician to diagnose and treat using these medical and surgical procedures to alleviate disease, pain, and suffering. But with the advent of YNSA, one is able to very effectively and efficiently provide speedy pain relief while effectively balancing out the neurophysiological abnormalities present with just a few needles placed correctly in the scalp. YNSA utilization with thoughtful consideration can be further enhanced by the practitioner's knowledge, skill, and ability in other macroacupuncture systems: TCM, French Energetics, and Five Phase acupuncture.

YNSA may be used as the primary treatment in neurological dysfunctions (i.e., pain, neuralgia, neuropathies, neuritis, and/or somatic dysfunction); however, the best results occur when YNSA is used in conjunction with orthodox medical, osteopathic, and/or chiropractic care. Cases treated with YNSA include post-CVA, paralysis, aphasia, cerebral palsy, sciatica, low back pain, herniated disc pain, spinal radiculopathy, painful spinal stenosis, tinnitus, arthritic pain, fibromyalgia, and medical conditions such as diabetes mellitus, hypothyroidism, menopause, dysmenorrhea, and other acute or recurrent painful conditions.

Summary

YNSA is a complete microsystem of the scalp acupuncture using Basic (anatomical) and Ypsilon (channel) points to affect the entire person. Toshikatsu Yamamoto, MD, PhD, discovered and developed this system in 1973. Basic and Ypsilon points found in the front of the head are called yin and the back of the head are called yang. Ypsilon points on the lateral side of the head in front of the auricle are called yin, and behind the auricle are called yang. Yin and yang are further divided into Yin of YIN, Yin of YANG, Yang of YIN, and Yang of YANG. YNSA is not like traditional CSA in that YNSA has a different somatotope, whereas CSA primarily uses representative areas on the scalp to stimulate the cerebral cortex for certain diseases. As in the auricular microsystem, YNSA has four phases. These four Ypsilon phases are defined as Yin of YIN, Yin of YANG, Yang of YIN, and Yang of YANG, which correlate with disease progression. YNSA may be used for a wide variety of medical and surgical conditions. It is not a substitute for surgical treatment of many anatomical pathological conditions. It may be used as a primary or secondary treatment for medical conditions. It has its best utilization in musculoskeletal and neurological conditions of pain and/or dysfunction. YNSA may be used in conjunction with other orthodox, standard medical and surgical treatments as a complementary treatment system.

乾 ䷀ 乾 ***Qián***

The Way of Initiating – Heaven Above, Heaven Below

"The way of the Initiating is change and transformation
So that each being obtains its true nature and destiny
And the union of great harmony is preserved.
This is what is favorable and upright."[12]

References

Additional references are available on p. 148. Acupoint schema and charts are found on p. 144 f.

1. Unschuld PU. Medicine in China: A History of Ideas. Berkeley, CA: University of California Press; 1985: 283
2. Oleson T. Auriculotherapy Manual: Chinese and Western Systems of Ear Acupuncture. Edinburgh: Churchill Livingstone; 1996: 11
3. Oleson T. Auriculotherapy Manual: Chinese and Western Systems of Ear Acupuncture. Edinburgh: Churchill Livingstone; 1996: 18–23
4. Bouevitch V. Microacupuncture systems as fractals of the human body. The Web-Journal of Acupuncture. 1996. Available at: http://med-vetacupuncture.org/english/articles/micros.html. Accessed November 26, 2009
5. Bensky D, O'Connor J. Acupuncture: A Comprehensive Text. Chicago: Eastland Press; 1981: 472
6. Oleson T. Auriculotherapy Manual: Chinese and Western Systems of Ear Acupuncture. Edinburgh: Churchill Livingstone; 1996: 165–270
7. Bensky D, O'Connor J. Acupuncture: A Comprehensive Text. Chicago, IL: Eastland Press; 1981: 473
8. Bensky D, O'Connor J. Acupuncture: A Comprehensive Text. Chicago, IL: Eastland Press; 1981: 501
9. Yamamoto T, Yamamoto H. Yamamoto New Scalp Acupuncture (YNSA). Tokyo, Japan: Axel Springer Japan Publishing, Inc.; 1998: 17
10. Bensky D, O'Connor J. Acupuncture: A Comprehensive Text. Chicago: Eastland Press; 1981: 497,498
11. Stux G, Pomerantz B. Basics of Acupuncture. 5th ed. Berlin, Germany: Springer; 1998: 7–23
12. Huang A. The Complete I Ching. Rochester, VT: Inner Traditions; 1998: 24

2

Traditional Chinese Medicine (TCM) and YNSA Theory

In the distant past lived the Yellow Emperor Huang Di. When he was born his spirit [was already characterized by an] all-pervading magic force. When still an infant he could already speak. In his youth he demonstrated a keen perceptive faculty. When he reached maturity his character was marked by a deep earnestness. When he reached adulthood he ascended to heaven. He put the following questions to the Celestial Master and spoke: "I have heard that the men of our ancient past experienced spring and autumn for one hundred years with no impairment of their ability to move and act. Today, however, it is so that men must limit their movements and actions after only half of a century. Have the times themselves changed or have men, that this [longevity] has been lost?"

To this Ch'i Po replied: "The men of antiquity understood the tao. *[They therefore strove to adapt their existence to] the rules of the* yin *and* yang *[duality] and to live in harmony…"*[1] *Huang-di Nei-jing Su-wen*

Chinese acupuncture theory. Since 200 BCE, the Chinese have left traces of the unique therapeutic activity of Chinese medicine. Ultimately they devised a system of life and health based on energetic and physiologic functions as represented through a network of channels pertaining to the flow of *qi*, blood, and moisture.

Needle's effect upon the scalp. The electrical action of the needle upon the biomagnetic field of the scalp is scientifically discussed.

Mechanisms of action. Several theories are discussed on how acupuncture works along with theories that are specific to scalp acupuncture. One such theory regarding the mechanical separation of the subcutaneous scalp tissues, resulting in the separation of microcalcifications, resulting in a change of electrical resistance is discussed.

Conclusions. From traditional Chinese medicine of acupuncture and moxibustion to YNSA, the highly skilled acupuncturist is touching *qi*, affecting the patient's electromagnetic field through the needle thereby influencing, promoting harmony and health.

This chapter discusses the great traditions of Oriental Medicine (OM), particularly as it originated in China. While it is true that Dr. Yamamoto is Japanese, knowledge of Oriental medicine is not required to perform YNSA, nevertheless, a basic understanding of the roots, philosophy, and terminology of Oriental medicine is quite helpful. Oriental medicine is based on Chinese medicine and the medical arts of Korea, Japan, and other Far Eastern lands which developed from it.

The roots of Chinese medicine go all the way back to the ancient texts including *Huang Di Nei Jing, Su Wen, Ling Shu, Nan Jing,* and *Zhen Jiu Jia Yi.* The premedical text that is presented at the end of each chapter throughout this book is the *I Ching,* the book of changes. The *I Ching* is a philosophical text that provides a contextual appreciation of ancient Chinese philosophical thought from which Oriental medicine and acupuncture sprang.

Eastern and Western Theories of Medicine

For centuries Western (Occidental) and Eastern (Oriental) thought were diametrically opposite. The Western physician approaches the patient from a very different cultural perspective than the Eastern physician. The Western physician starts with patients presenting symptoms and then theorizes using Cartesian and linear thinking based on Newtonian physics to search for the underlining mechanism. This Newtonian way of looking at life causes the Western physician to look for the exact material, biochemical, or physiological cause of the symptoms—whether they are from trauma or other external or internal pathological causes—and invent a label for the disease, a name. This name is given to a specific constilation of physical signs, symptoms, and related tests and/or microorganisms. The best Western physician is trained to be analytical and linear in thinking, with the physician trapped into searching for a specific cause, ideally a single cause and its related effect, as exemplified by the gold standard of Western scientific medical research—the randomized, controlled, matched, double-blind, single or double crossover research study. This line of thought continues with the search for the "magic bullet," the single intervention, drug, surgery, or procedure to stop or reverse the symptom if not the disease.

The Eastern physician approaches the patient from a global, contextual, organic perspective using both Quantum and Newtonian thought. This physician views patients from a perspective of looking for harmony within their environment and noting their presenting disharmony or symptom. The Eastern physician does this by looking at patients' biographical, psychological, emotional, and biological states in addition to their the symptoms. The Eastern physician identifies health first and then interweaves a description of characteristics and current symptomology to identify "dysharmonies," deviation(s) from perfect health. This poetic, yet workable, description of the patient engenders a prescription or a formula for therapeutic action based on the central Chinese concepts of systematic correspondences.[2]

The difference can be described as the following—The West asks the question, What X is causing Y disease? The East asks, What is the relationship between X and Y? The West looks for the silver bullet to save a life, stop a symptom, or kill a germ. The East looks for dysharmony and tries to reconfigure the physiology and psychology to restore harmony, which is a definition of health.[3] Another way to sum it up is: The Western physician's thought process is linear, uniformly measured, and materialistic. The Eastern physician's thought process is quantum mechanical, individually assessed, and vitalistic.

Chinese Principles and Terms

YNSA is a microsystem of acupuncture that uses a simple, yet complex, system of diagnostic and treatment protocols. Knowledge of OM or Traditional Chinese Medicine (TCM) acupuncture theory and practice is very helpful but not required to practice YNSA. For those readers without any TCM knowledge, the following Chinese principles and terms are given.

In the 16th century, the Jesuits returned to Europe from China with a new medical treatment in Latin called *acus punctura* or acupuncture, but until recently in North America acupuncture was not widely accepted because it clashed with the accepted paradigms of Western medicine.[4] China, the prevailing philosophical constructs in which acupuncture and TCM were developed was based on holistic patterns, a causal relationship, nonlinear logic, and nonreductionistic phenomenology. By contrast, Western medicine is based on reductionistic scientific theories and causality. Chinese Taoism had a disdain for explanatory theories and chose instead to merely observe phenomena to maintain harmony with nature.[5]

The Chinese physician/philosophers before 200 BCE had been involved in defining humanity's place on the earth and under heaven. The Chinese philosophers saw humans as a connection between the terrestrial (earthly) and the ethereal (heavenly). Because they saw humans as the center of the universe (their world), humans were viewed as the connection between heaven and earth, with both forces having an influence upon human existence. This influence could be either beneficial or detrimental to health. The philosophers devised the following principles:

- One energy of life: *qi*
- Two basic polarities: *yin* and *yang*
- Three fluids: *qi*, blood, and moisture
- Four seasons: winter, spring, summer, and autumn
- Five phases: wood, fire, earth, metal, and water
- Six climates of nature: cold, summer heat, fire, wind, damp, and dryness
- Seven emotions; joy, anger, anxiety, concentration, grief, fear, fright
- Eight bodily fluids: Life Energy (*qi*), Nourishing Qi (*ying qi*), Protecting Qi (*wei qi*), Blood (*xue*), Essence (*jing*), Semen (*jing*), Spirit (*shen*), Clear Fluid (*jin*), Thick Fluid (*ye*).

Qi 气

Qi (pronounced chee) is the vital energy and is symbolized by two parts of the ideogram: *qi*, for air and for breathing, and *mi*, for grain as the origin of nutrition.[6] *Qi* signifies movement, something on the order of energy, the energy of life. *Qi* has two unique aspects. First, and most importantly, it is thought of as matter without form. Second, it is a term for the functional active state of the body. In *The Yellow Emperor's Classic of Internal Medicine (Huang Di Nei Jing)* first published in 100 BCE there are many keys to OM thought. In it the *Su Wen*, known as *Simple Questions*, chapter 25, states, "a human being results from the *qi* of heaven and earth ... the union of heaven and earth is called human being." In the classic of difficulties, it says, "*qi* is the root of a human being." There are two particular aspects of *qi* that are relevant to medicine: (1) *qi* is an energy that manifests simultaneously on the physical and spiritual level and (2) *qi* is in a constant state of flux; when *qi* condenses, energy transforms and accumulates into physical shape.

When acupuncture physicians attempt to make a diagnosis, they are evaluating the presence and character of *qi* in all its many states. When acupuncture is used, *qi* is said to be obtained with the needle and then manipulated. The act of grabbing the *qi* and obtaining it with a needle is called *de qi*.

In Chinese medicine, there are several types of *qi*. One is source *qi*. It is the basal energy of the body formed from the essence of the kidneys, the nutrients absorbed from food, and the energy absorbed by the lungs from the air. Source *qi* is manifested in various ways. First, there is organ *qi*, which is the physiological activity and functions of each organ. Second, is the channel or channel *qi*, which is the transportive and moving function of the channels. Third, is nourishing *qi*, which is the *qi* that moves with the blood. Its functions are transforming blood, creating blood, and helping the blood nourish the tissues of the body. Fourth, is protective *qi*, which is the *qi* that travels outside the channels. Protective *qi* warms the organs and travels subcutaneously between the skin and the muscle to regulate the opening and closing of pores. The fifth and final *qi* is the ancestral *qi*, the *qi* that collects in the chest. The center point is Ren-17 (*chan zhong*).

"*Qi* may be understood as a matterless forcefield on which matter is constructed, organized, expressed, directed, and affected. *Qi* creates and 'moves' or directs matter; acupuncture stimulates or otherwise manipulates that *qi* or matterless forcefield."[7]

The energy of life, *qi*, is the fundamental concept of Chinese thought. This electromagnetic force has a pervasive and diffusive influence on the physiology and function of each person. There are various types of *qi*; however, there is ultimately only one *qi*, merely manifesting itself in different forms in various parts of the body and

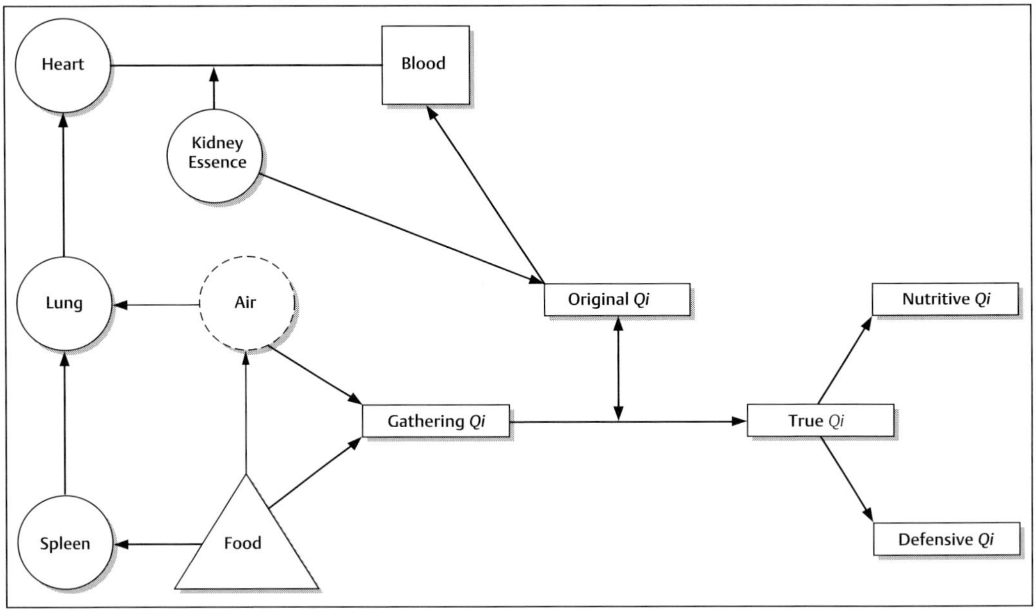

Figure 2–1 Development of *qi* and blood.

at various stages of development. The ancient text of the *Ling Shu* describes true *qi*: *True* Qi *is a combination of what is received from the heavens and the* Qi *of water and food. It permeates the whole body. Qi* changes its form according to its location and function. *Zhangshi Leijing* further tells us that: *True* Qi *is the original* Qi. Qi *from heaven is received through the nose and controlled by the windpipe;* Qi *from food and water enters the stomach and is controlled by the gullet. That which nourishes the unborn is the* Qi *of the former heaven (pre-natal); that which fills the (new)born is called the* qi *of the latter heaven (post-natal).* Original *Qi* is in the lower burner, which is below the navel and above the pubic synthesis. Original *Qi* nourishes the kidneys.[8]

A more complete description of how *qi* is transformed is as follows. Original *Qi* is nothing but essence in the form of *qi* rather than fluid and it relies on nourishment from the postheaven essence. Its functions are a dynamic motive force that arouses and moves the functional activity of all organs. Original *Qi* is the basis for kidney *qi*. Original *Qi* occupies the acupuncture source points and dwells between the two kidneys below the umbilicus and posterior to the gate of vitality Du-4 (*ming men*). It acts as an agent of change in the transformation of Gathering *Qi* into True *Qi*. It also facilitates the transformation of Food *Qi* into blood. Food *Qi* comes from the middle burner (stomach, spleen, and small intestine) and it rises to the chest where it combines with the air from the lungs and forms the Gathering *Qi*, also called Essential *Qi*. True *Qi* is the last stage of transformational *Qi* where Gathering *Qi* is transformed under the catalytic action of Original *Qi*. True *Qi* is the final stage of the process of refinement and transformation where *qi* circulates in the channels and nourishes the organs.

True Qi becomes one of two different forms—Nutritive *Qi* and Defensive *Qi*. Nutritive *Qi* is closely related to the blood and flows in the blood vessels, following the course of the channels. Defensive *Qi* is in a *yang* relationship to Nutritive *Qi*. It is on the exterior and protects the body from attack by external pathogenic physical factors such as wind, cold, heat, and damp. Defensive *Qi* has its root in the lower burner, the kidneys, and is nourished by the middle burner, stomach, and spleen. It spreads outwards in the upper burner, the lungs. Defensive *Qi* circulates 50 times in a 24-hour cycle, see **Figure 2–1**.

The basic functions of *qi* are transforming, transporting, holding, raising, protecting, and warming. The spleen transforms food into food *qi*, kidney *qi* transforms the fluids, the bladder *qi* transforms urine, and the heart *qi* transforms food *qi* into the blood. Principle transportation duties of *qi* occur with the spleen *qi* transporting the food *qi*, and the lung *qi* transporting the fluids to the skin.

The direction of movement of *qi* is as follows: the kidney *qi* transports the *qi* upward, the liver *qi* transports the *qi* in all directions, and the lung *qi* transports *qi* downward. The function of controlling fluids and the blood in the blood vessels is done by the spleen *qi*. The kidney *qi* and bladder *qi* hold the urine. The lung *qi* holds the sweat. The spleen *qi* and the kidney *qi* rise upward while the lung *qi* protects the body from external pathogens. Both the spleen *yang* and kidney *yang* functions are to warm the body.[9]

The Su Wen further describes *qi* on earth as follows: That which was from the beginning in heaven is *Qi*; on earth it becomes visible as form; *Qi* and form interact, give birth to the myriad things. The qi flows through these vessels called channels. Yijiang Jingyi tells us that "the channels are the paths of the transforming action of *Qi* in the solid and hollow organs."[10] *Qi* is a *yang* characteristic that is the basis of all bodily energy.

Blood 血

In Chinese medicine, blood, or *xue*, is composed of two ideograms; *chu* for a drop, and *min* for a vessel.[11] *Xue* or blood is more than just the red blood cells and liquid that circulate throughout the body; it is also regarded as a force in OM and has a level of activity in the body that is involved in the sensitivity of the sense organs. Traditionally, it is said that blood is manufactured in the middle burner using *qi* derived from food digested by the spleen, *gu qi*, or food *qi*, and from the air in the lungs, *zong qi*, or air *qi*. Blood is a *yin* substance.

Essence 精

Essence, called *jing*, is a *yin* characteristic that is the basis for all growth, development, and sexuality. *Jing* is composed of two ideograms: *mi* for grain and *quing* for fresh or young. The young grain symbolizes the essence of life.[11] The traditional Chinese medical books describe *jing* in three different contexts with slightly different meanings. Preheaven essence or *jing* is the blending of the sexual energies of male and female to conceive a human being. Postheaven essence or *jing* is refined and extracted from food and fluids by the stomach and spleen after birth. Kidney essence or *jing* derives from both pre- and postheaven essence and determines growth, reproductive development, sexual maturation, conception, and pregnancy.

The difference between essence and *qi* within the human body is that *qi* is formed after birth and essence or *jing* is derived from the parents. *Qi* is energy-like. Essence is fluid-like. *Qi* is everywhere and essence resides mostly in the kidneys. *Qi* can easily be replenished on a dayto-day basis. Essence is replenished only with great difficulty, if at all. *Qi* flows in short cycles—some yearly, some monthly, and some daily—while a few are even shorter, whereas essence flows in 6-year cycles for women and 8-year cycles for men. *Qi* moves and changes quickly from moment to moment, whereas essence changes slowly and gradually over decades. Congenital essence or *jing* can never be replaced. Essence or *jing* may also be used narrowly to mean semen.

Spirit 神

Shen means spirit, psychic energy, reasoning ability, and consciousness. The original means of *shen* in ancient China, in the cultural context of ancestor worship, was communication between humans and gods by way of spirits. The *shen* consists of two ideograms: *shi*, which means to make known and *shen*, which means to report. The commentator of the *Huai Tzu* says, "*Jing* is the *qi* of the person" and "*shen* is the protective nature of the person."[12] The *Su Wen* says, "if the shen is damaged or leaves, we cannot cure the disease."[12] The *Ling Shu* describes the continuum of *jing* and *shen* thus, "when the two *shen* meet, form is created. Before the form is created, this is *Jing*. When the two *Jing* meet, shen is formed." The *I Ching* describes *jing* and *shen* as "*Jing* creates the form" when "*Yin-Yang* cannot be measured, it is called *Shen*." Finally, the *Ling Shu* and the *Su Wen* tells us where the *jing* and the *shen* are stored. "*Jing* is stored in the kidneys" and "*Shen* is stored in the heart."[12] Spirit, or *shen*, is a *yang* characteristic that is the force behind one's mental state and actions.[13] *Beji yang* spirit is received from heaven and is manifested in consciousness and thought.

Fluid

Fluids of the body include sweat, urine, tears, saliva, and other secretions. They are either thin, *jin*, or thick, *ye* (*yang* or *yin*, respectively). The thin fluid moistens the muscles, skin, flesh, and membranes. The thick fluid moistens the inner organs and brain. Fluids are a *yin* characteristic.

Yin/Yang

The Chinese believed that the beginning of the world was a formless, indivisible whole. For life to develop, the unity had to become a duality, and from this idea came the concept of complementary opposites, which they called *yin* and *yang*. This duality is pervasive in Chinese life, art, literature, philosophy, and medicine.

Yang 阳

This *yin* and *yang* concept is at the cornerstone of Chinese and Oriental thought. *Yang* consists of two ideograms: *fu* is for hill and *yang* is for brightness, expansiveness. *Yang* is the sunny side of the hill.

Yin 阴

Yin consists of two ideograms: *jin* is for now or present and *yun* is for clouds. *Yin* is the shady side of the hill.[14]

The *Taiji* or great polarity is a symbol of *yin* and *yang* as seen in **Figure 2–2**. *Yin* and *yang* are emblems of the fundamental duality within Chinese medicine and describe the universe. The color black in the *Taiji* signifies *yin* and white signifies *yang*. These two colors coil around, fade into, and penetrate each other. Both *yin* and *yang* are necessary for the whole to exist. This *yin–yang* concept is projected to all levels of the universe and a system of correspondences. *Yin* and *yang* are complementary. They are not contradictory. Nor is one good and the other bad. It is the harmony between them that is sought and the avoidance of imbalance that provides health and life. To be able to distinguish between the *yin* and *yang* quality of a person's constitution or illness is an important step in the process of synthesizing the necessity for proper treatment using traditional Chinese medicine and YNSA.

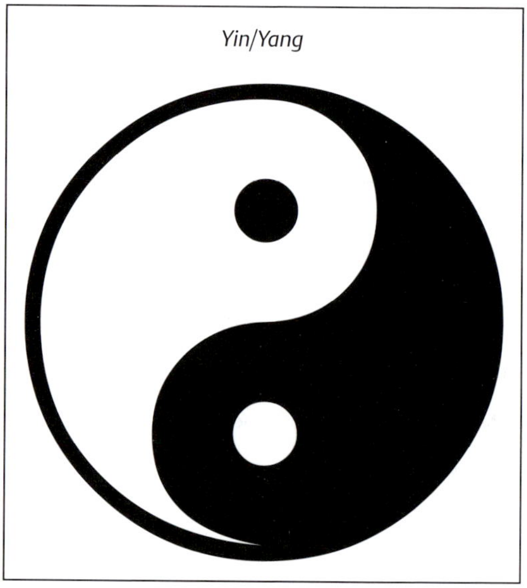

Figure 2–2 The *Yin/yang* symbol *Taijitu* (literally "diagram of the supreme ultimate").

The *yin* and *yang* correspondences are seen in medical conditions. **Table 2–1** lists correspondences for the cosmos.

Yin

- Inferior, anterior medial surface, structure, ventral surface, interior, front, lower section, bones, inner organs, blood, inhibition, vacuity, solid organs

Yang

- Superior, posterior lateral surface, function of a structure, dorsal surface, exterior, back, upper section, skin, outer organs, qi, stimulation, repletion, hollow organs

Yin and *yang* are relative terms. It is important to understand that what is *yin* in relation to one thing may be *yang* in relation to another.[13] *Yin* and *yang* must succeed one another so that in a *yin* condition the corresponding *yang* state can be

Table 2–1 *Yin/yang* cosmos correspondences

Yin	*Yang*
Earth	Heaven
Female	Male
Night	Day
Moon	Sun
Low	High
Heaviness	Lightness
Matter	Energy
Falling tendency	Rising tendency
Moving inward	Moving outward
Flat	Round
West	East
North	South
Right	Left
Relative stasis	Clear action
Quiet	Active

foretold and vice versa. The qualities of *yin* and *yang* are relative and not absolute.

The *Su Wen* best describes *yin* and *yang* the way we use it in YNSA: "There is *yin* within YIN and *yang* within YANG. From dawn till noon, the *yang* of heaven is within the YANG; from noon till dusk the *yin* of heaven is within the YANG; from dusk till midnight the *yin* of heaven is within the YIN; from midnight till dawn the *yang* of heaven is within the YIN."[15] We describe all Basic and Ypsilon points in *yin* or *yang* terms and then further divide YIN into *yin* or *yang* and YANG is also divided into *yin* or *yang*.

Yin and *yang* are two phases of a cyclical movement, alternating between day and night. The sun is in the heaven, therefore the heaven is *yang* and the earth is *yin*. The ancient Chinese farmers thought heaven was a round vault and the earth was flat, therefore *yang* is round and *yin* is square. Because the sun rises in the east and sets in the west, the east is *yang* and the west is *yin*. The directions are further divided by Chinese tradition.

In Chinese imperial ceremonies it is quoted, "the emperor face south towards the subjects who face north."[16] The emperor thus opened himself up to see the influence of heaven *yang* and south. South is, therefore, like heaven at the top, *yang*. North is, therefore, like earth at the bottom, *yin*. By facing south, the emperor identifies his left with the east and his right with the west. Thus, left corresponds to *yang* and right to *yin*.

In the *Su Wen*, it says, "east represents *yang*, west represents *yin*, in the west and in the north there is a deficiency of heaven hence the left ear and eyes hear and see better than the right, in the east and south there is deficiency of earth hence the right hand and foot are stronger than the left." The second chapter of *Su Wen* says: "Heaven is the accumulation of *yang* and earth is the accumulation of *yin*." Thus, in the purest and more rarified form, *yang* is totally immaterial and corresponds to pure energy and *yin* in its coarsest and densest form is totally material and corresponds to matter. Again in chapter 2 of *Su Wen*, "*yin* is quiet and *yang* is active. *Yang* gives life and *yin* makes it grow. *Yang* is transformed into *qi* and *yin* is transformed into material life."

There are four main aspects of *yin* and *yang* in their relationship. First, *yin* and *yang* are opposite stages of each other's cycle. However, the opposition is relative and not absolute in so far as nothing is totally *yin* or totally *yang*. The second aspect is the interdependence of *yin* and *yang*. Although they are opposites, one cannot exist without the other. Everything contains opposite forces that are mutually exclusive but, at the same time, are dependent upon each other. The third aspect in the *yin/yang* relationship is that they are in a constant state of dynamic balance, which is maintained by a continuous adjustment of the relative values of *yin* and *yang*. The fourth aspect of their relationship is that *yin* and *yang* are not static. They actually transform into each other. *Yin* can change into *yang* and *yang* can change into *yin*.

Yin/Yang Relationship

- Opposites
- Interdependent
- In dynamic balance
- Transformation

Therapeutic Purpose of Acupuncture and Chinese Medical Thought

The application of *yin* and *yang* toward medicine is that every acupuncture treatment is aimed at one of the four stages: to tonify or strengthen *yang* when a vacuity is found, to tonify or strengthen *yin* when a vacuity is found, to disperse or purge *yang* repletion when found, or to disperse or purge *yin* repletion when it is found.

As a general rule, the following characteristics of various body structures are *yang*: the superior, exterior, posterior lateral surface, the back, and the function of a structure. The following body structures are *yin*: inferior, interior, anterior medial surface, front, and structure. The head is the one place where all *yang* channels either begin or end; they meet and flow into each other in the head.

Five Phases

Wu Xing 五行

According to Chinese philosophy, the transformation of life is accomplished in the Five Phases or Five Elements (**Fig. 2–3**) also known as *wu xing*. *Wu* is the ideogram for five and *xing* means to go, the journey, and the change. Its ideogram is composed of *chi*, which means small step and *chu*, which means to go to.[14]

The late professor J.R. Worsley, in *Classical Five Element Acupuncture: The Five Elements and the Officials* states, "Every living thing and every person on the planet is a unique embodiment and combination of the five elements."[17] "The five elements express and embody the aspects of this change and movement within the *qi* energy. Each element describes a particular phase of its movement, the particular qualities that belong to that part of its changing pattern. Together the elements help us to understand the process of dynamic harmony and balance in the whole system of energy. Through this they give us the insight, which allows us to promote by our system of medicine. When we look at the individual elements, therefore, we always have to keep in

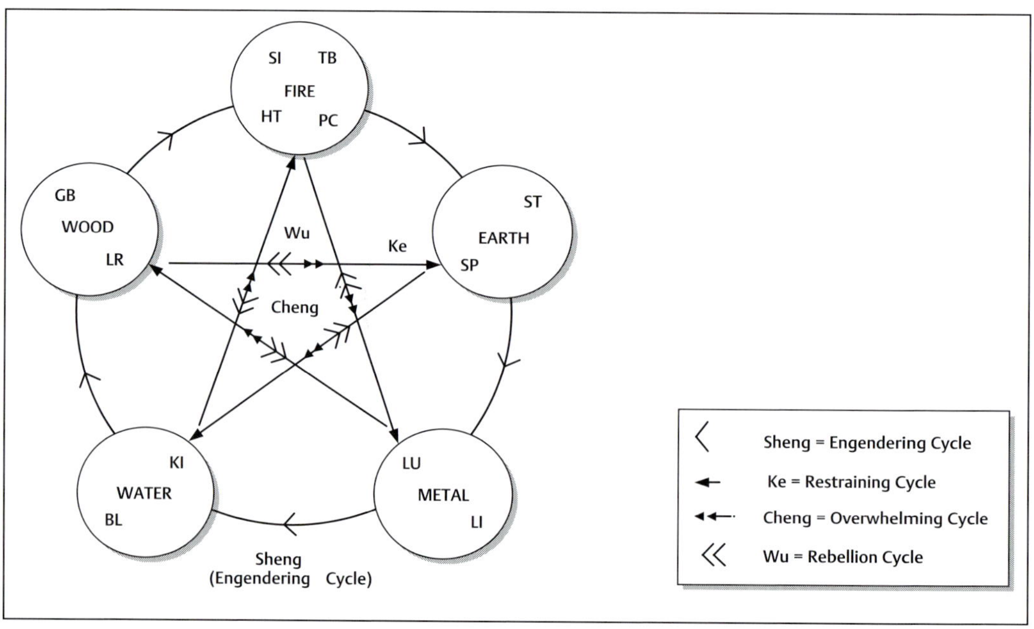

Figure 2–3 Five phase pentagram.

our minds that we are looking at parts of a much larger picture. As practitioners of acupuncture who treat the whole person, this must be one of most important guiding principles."[17]

The Five Phase system of acupuncture is based on the ancient Chinese medical and premedical texts including *Huang Di Nei Jing, Su Wen, Ling Shu, Nan Jing,* and *Zhen Jiu Jia Yi Jing*. There is a strong resemblance between the phase name in the Chinese translations of fire, earth, metal, water, and wood and the four phases of the Greco-European thought of fire, earth, water, and air. This Five Phase approach is a very complete system of correspondences, providing excellent reasoning and methodology for a complete diagnosis and treatment.

The earliest reference to Five Phases can be seen in *Shu Ching*, a book on political philosophy circulated between the 10th and 5th centuries BCE. Similar information can be found in the *Li Chi*, or the Book of Rights, as early as the 5th century BCE and in the *Guan Dzu*, a book of philosophy, dating back to the 4th century BCE. The Five Phase concept's first known application to the body and to medicine was in the *Su Wen* written ~100 BCE. Five Phases also appeared in the *Ling Shu* and in the most complete and profound way in the *Nan Jing*. Here, the development of Five Phase theories and correspondences was complete. In the *Nan Jing*, the development and synthesis of cycles, correspondences, and theories were made realizing the limitations of these ideas. As Kiiko Matsumoto and Stephen Birch point out in their book, *Five Elements and Ten Stems*, "the Five Element system was not seen as a hard and fast doctrine but rather a problem solving device."[18]

The Five Phases are described as fire, water, wood, metal, and earth. Fire relates directly to heart (HT), small intestine (SI), pericardium (PC), and triple burner (TB). Water relates directly to the kidney (KI) and bladder (BL). Wood relates directly to the liver (LR) and gall bladder (GB). Metal relates directly to the lung (LU) and large intestine (LI). Earth relates directly to spleen (SP) and stomach (ST). In **Table 2–2**, each phase has *yin* and *yang* components, also known as the *zang* and *fu* organs.

Table 2–2 (*Zang*) *Yin–Yang* (*Fu*) organs

Yin (Zang) 脏	*Yang (Fu)* 腑
HT	SI
KI	BL
PC	TB
LR	GB
LU	LI
SP	ST

Fu are *yang* organs such as gall bladder, small intestine, stomach, large intestine, and bladder. *Fu* organs are considered hollow organs. The *fu* ideogram is composed of two parts: *rou* for flesh and *fu* for prefecture, or the official residence. *Fu* organs act as governing authorities, influencing the connecting *yin* organs. The *zang* organs are *yin* organs such as the liver, heart, spleen, lung, and kidney. The *zang* organs, by tradition, are described as storing the vital energy. *Zang* organs are considered solid organs.[12] *Zang* consists of two ideograms: *rou*, which means flesh, and *zang*, which is to hide, to pressure, and to store.

Each element or phase is a symbol that represents a category of related functions and qualities, as shown in **Table 2–3**. Wood is associated with active functions such as growing and increasing. Fire is associated with functions that have reached their maximum state. Metal relates to functions that are declining. Water represents the functions that have reached a maximum state of decline. Earth represents balance and neutrality. Earth acts as a buffer between the other four phases. These five phases act as generic categories for the classification of all phenomena; from colors and sounds to orders, tastes, emotions, animals, destinies, planets, and all things known in the cosmos.

The *Shang Shu* says, "The five elements are water, fire, wood, metal, and earth. Water moistens downwards, fire flares upwards, wood can be bent and straightened, metal can be molded and hardened, earth permits sowing, growing, and reaping that which soaks and descends, 'water' is salty. That which blazes upwards 'fire' is bitter, that which can be bent and straightened 'wood' is sour, that which can be molded and become hard 'metal' is pungent, that which permits sowing and reaping 'earth' is sweet."

These five phases also represent directions of movement of natural phenomena, see **Table 2–4**.

Table 2–3 Human five phase table

Element/ Phase	*Yin/Yang*	Channel/ Official	Symbol	Attributes	Color	Sound	Odors	Bowel	Orifice	Sense	Tissue
WOOD	*Yang*	Gall bladder	**GB**	Decision making, Judge	Green	Shouting	Greasy/ Rancid	Gall bladder	Eye	Sight	Muscles
	Yin	Liver	**LR**	Strategic planning, Architect							
FIRE	*Yang*	Small intes-tine	**SI**	Screener, Private secretary	Red	Laughing	Burnt/ Scorched	Small intes-tine,	The 7 orifices	Taste	Blood vessels
	Yin	Heart	**HT**	Life of the party				Triple burner			
	Yang	Triple burner	**TB**	Supreme controller							
	Yin	Pericardium	**PC**	Building heating engineer, Ambassador							
EARTH	*Yang*	Stomach	**ST**	Supply sergeant,	Yellow	Singing	Sweet/ Fragrant	Stomach	Mouth	Touch	Flesh
	Yin	Spleen	**SP**	Mother, Transportation manager							
METAL	*Yang*	Large intes-tine	**LI**	Garbage man Priest/pastor,	White	Weeping	Rank/ Rotten	Large intes-tine	Nose	Smell	Skin
	Yin	Lung	**LU**	Father							
WATER	*Yang*	Bladder	**BL**	Banker	Blue/ Black	Groaning	Putrid/ Musty	Bladder	Ear, Urinary meatus, Rectum	Hearing	Bone
	Yin	Kidney	**KI**	Wise grandmother							

Element/ Phase	Taste	Voice	Sense Organ	Power	Body Types	Fortifies	Fluids	Tone	Number	Metal	Mythical Animal
WOOD	Sour	Square	Eyes	Birth	Pointed, small hands	Ligaments	Tears	Jiao = 3rd	8	Tin	Dragon
FIRE	Bitter	Long, harmonize	Tongue	Mature	Large, strong hands	Arteries	Sweat	Zhi = 4th	7	Iron	Sun
EARTH	Sweet	Big, moderate	Mouth	Decrease	Triangular features	Muscles	Sticky saliva	Gong = 1st	5	Lead	Bird
METAL	Pungent	Loud, sobbing	Nose	Balance	Round features	Skin and hair	Runny nose	Shang = 2nd	9	Copper	Tiger
WATER	Salty	Quiet	Ears	Emphasis	Tall, slender	Bones	Watery saliva	Yu = 5th	6	Mercury	Moon or tortoise

Table 2–4 Physical five phase table

Element/Phase	*Yin/Yang*	Channel	Symbol	Time of Day	Directions	Season	Climate	Grains	Meat	Fruit	Plant
WOOD	*Yang*	Gall bladder	**GB**	11pm–1 am	East	Spring	Wind	Wheat	Chicken	Plum	Pine tree
	Yin	Liver	**LR**	1 am–3 am							
FIRE	*Yang*	Small intestine	**SI**	1 pm–3 pm	South	Summer	Heat	Millet flour	Sheep	Apricot	Iris flower
	Yin	Heart	**HT**	11 am–1pm							
FIRE	*Yang*	Triple burner	**TB**	9 pm–11pm	South	Summer	Heat	Millet flour	Sheep	Apricot	Iris flower
	Yin	Pericardium	**PC**	7 pm–9 pm							
EARTH	*Yang*	Stomach	**ST**	7 am–9 am	Center	Late summer	Humidity	Millet	Cow	Date	Bermuda grass
	Yin	Spleen	**SP**	9 am–11am							
METAL	*Yang*	Large intestine	**LI**	5 am–7 am	West	Autumn	Dryness	Rice	Horse	Peach	Oak tree
	Yin	Lung	**LU**	3 am–5 am							
WATER	*Yang*	Bladder	**BL**	3 pm–5 pm	North	Winter	Cold	Bean	Pig	Chestnut	Barrow cactus
	Yin	Kidney	**KI**	5 pm–7 pm							

Table 2–5 Five element key words table[19]

Wood	Fire	Earth	Metall	Water
Vision	Understanding	Nourishing	Quality	Reserves
Birth	Fullness	Ingest	Inspiration	Determination
Growth	Joy	Assimilate	Death	Endurance
Structure	Warmth	Distribute	Essence Distilled	Quiet
Flexible	Maturity	Security	Respect	Elusive
Purpose	Spirit	Stability	Letting Go	Impenetrable
Movement	Love	Balance	Divine	Still
Hope	Openness	Mother	Father	Fear

Table 2–6 Engendering (*Sheng*) cycle

	Wood	Fire	Earth	Metal	Water
Child	Child of Water	Child of Wood	Child of Fire	Child of Earth	Child of Metal
Mother	Mother of Fire	Mother of Earth	Mother of Metal	Mother of Water	Mother of Wood

Wood represents expansive outward movement in all directions, whereas metal represents a contracted inward movement. Fire represents upward movement and water represents downward movement, whereas earth represents neutrality and stability.

Wood corresponds with the spring and birth. Fire corresponds to summer and is associated with growth. Metal corresponds with autumn and late harvest. Water corresponds to winter and storage. Earth corresponds to the late summer season and is associated with transformation.

Professor J.R. Worsley, the 20th century's leading Five Phase acupuncturist, in his text, *Classical Five-Element Acupuncture: The Five Elements and the Officials*, states the key words that would describe each of the five phases.[19] The one word that best describes wood is *vision*. The other words that would describe the patient when taking a history or diagnosing of a wood (causative factor) patient would be; *birth*, *growth*, *structure*, etcetera. Take a close look at **Table 2–5**, which summarizes these descriptive words nicely.

Five Phase Movement

Looking again at the Five Phase Pentagram (**Fig. 2–3**), the engendering, restraining, overwhelming, and rebellion cycles of the Five Phases are completely depicted. This first movement is called the engendering sequence or *Sheng* cycle, where one phase gives rise to the next phase. It is key in propagating life or *qi* through the channels. So the initial phase is called mother and gives birth or life to the next phase called child. Thus, wood (mother) generates fire (child), fire (mother) generates earth (child), earth (mother) generates metal (child), metal (mother) generates water (child), and water (mother) generates wood (child). So it is said that wood is the child of water and the mother of fire, see **Table 2–6**.

The restraining cycle, or *Ke* cycle, is the second movement whereby each phase controls another from being too replete. By controlling its corresponding phase, it promotes balance and harmony. Thus, wood controls the earth, earth controls the water, water controls the fire, fire controls the metal, and metal controls the wood, see **Table 2–7**. So, wood controls the earth but is also controlled by the metal. This restraining

Table 2–7 Restraining (*Ke*) cycle

Origin	Controlled
Wood	Earth
Earth	Water
Water	Fire
Fire	Metal
Metal	Wood

Table 2–8 Overwhelming (*Cheng*) cycle

Origin	Overactant
Wood	Earth
Earth	Water
Water	Fire
Fire	Metal
Metal	Wood

Table 2–9 Rebellion (*Wu*) cycle

Origin	Insultant
Fire	Water
Water	Earth
Earth	Wood
Wood	Metal
Metal	Fire

cycle is key in providing balance and harmony within the channels. The Five Phase model provides clinically useful patterns for identification of pathological relationships between the internal organs as well as psychological states.

The third action of movement of the Five Phases is the overwhelming, or *Cheng* cycle, as depicted in **Table 2–8**. The overwhelming cycle occurs in the same order as the restraining (*Ke*) cycle but is much more replete to the detriment of the recipient phase. When wood overacts on earth, earth becomes vacuous and unable to nurture metal. Metal is then unable, through the restraining (*Ke*) cycle, to control wood. Wood, then, becomes replete also, passing a more excessive overacting force upon the earth phase. In another case, when earth overacts on water, water is unable to nurture wood. Thus, wood is unable to control the earth phase and the cycle exacerbates and continues. When water overacts on fire, fire diminishes and is unable to control metal. Metal increases to foster even more water. When fire overacts on metal, metal is unable to control wood and unable to generate water. Then wood generates more fire, which overacts on metal and starts the cycle again. When metal overacts on wood, wood is unable to control earth and unable to support fire. Earth generates more metal and the cycle repeats.

The fourth movement—the rebellion, or *Wu* cycle—occurs in the reverse of the restraining (*Ke*) cycle, see **Table 2–9**. This back-up of energy is replete (excess) in imposing a deleterious effect upon its recipient phase. When fire dominates and insults the water, water diminishes. When water insults the earth, the earth diminishes. When earth insults the wood, the wood diminishes. When wood insults the metal, the metal diminishes.

The overwhelming (*Cheng*) and rebellion (*Wu*) cycles are a reflection of an imbalance or abnormal relationship among the Five Phases. For an illustration of these relationships among each Five Phases, see **Figs. 2–3** to **2–9**. This abnormal relationship over time produces disease.

Clinical Examples of Five Phase Movements

When the restraining (*Ke*) cycle gradually becomes replete to the point of being overwhelming (*Cheng* cycle), the relationship among the phases results in repletions. For example, when the liver (wood) becomes replete and controls or overacts on the stomach and spleen, it is said that the liver *qi* stagnates and invades the stomach impairing the function of rotting and ripening. The spleen is impaired in its function of transforming and transporting. It prevents the stomach *qi* from descending causing the symptom—nausea. This prevents the spleen *qi* from ascending, causing diarrhea. Another example is when the heart (fire) controls or overacts on the lungs. Heart fire can dry up the lung (metal) fluid

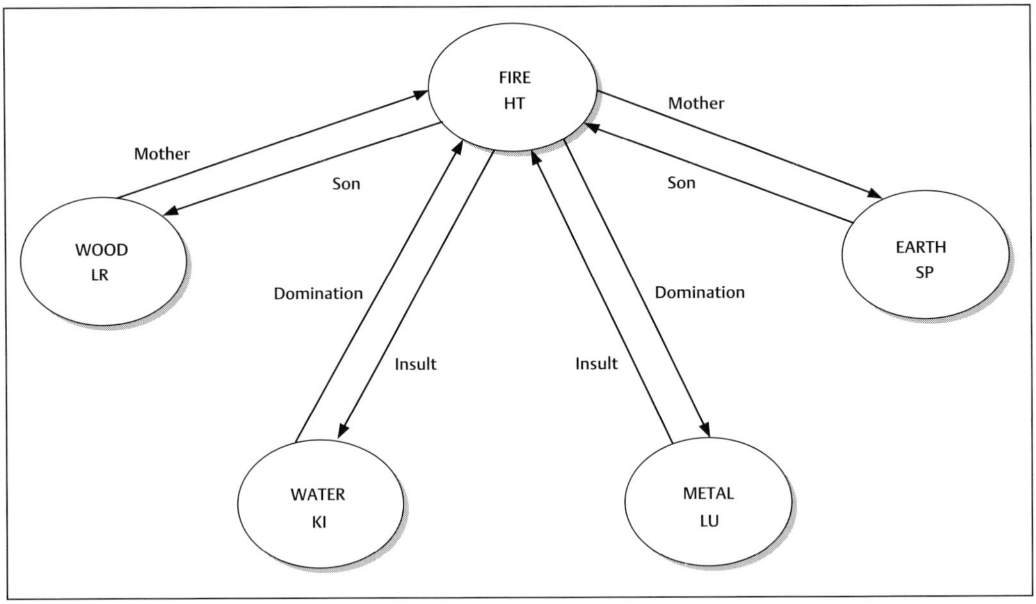

Figure 2–4 Fire complete movements.

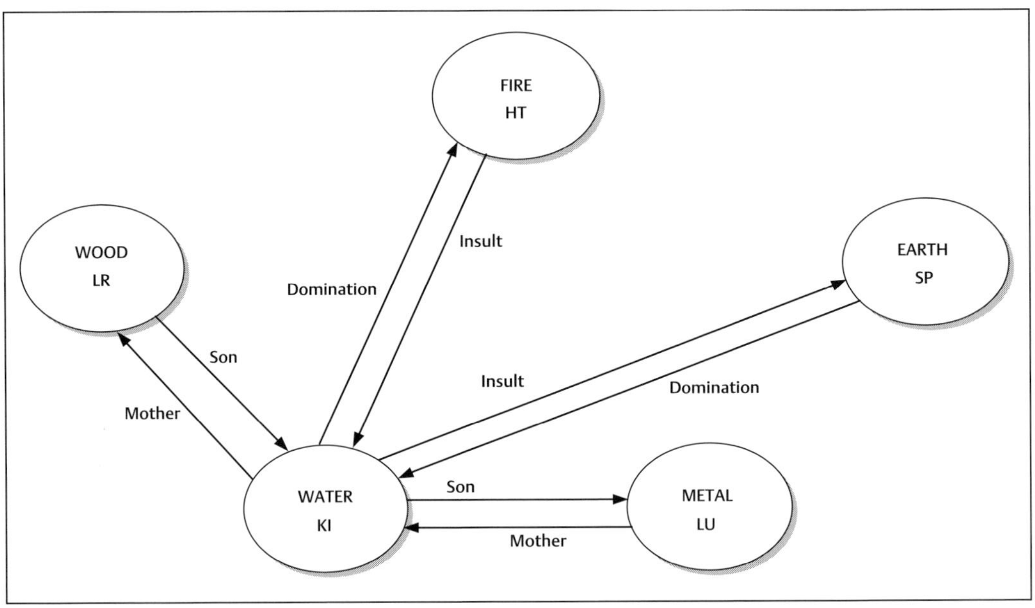

Figure 2–5 Water complete movements.

causing lung *yin* vacuity (deficient) with signs and symptoms of a dry, nonproductive cough, night sweating, red cheeks, and low-grade fever.

When the spleen (earth) overacts on the kidneys (water), the spleen holds dampness and this can obstruct the function of the kidney transformation and excretion of fluids, which may give rise to water retention, nausea, and possible urinary tract infections. When the lungs (metal) overact on the liver (wood), this is a case of lung vacuity triggering stagnation of the liver *qi*, which may lead to hay fever, tight cough with dif-

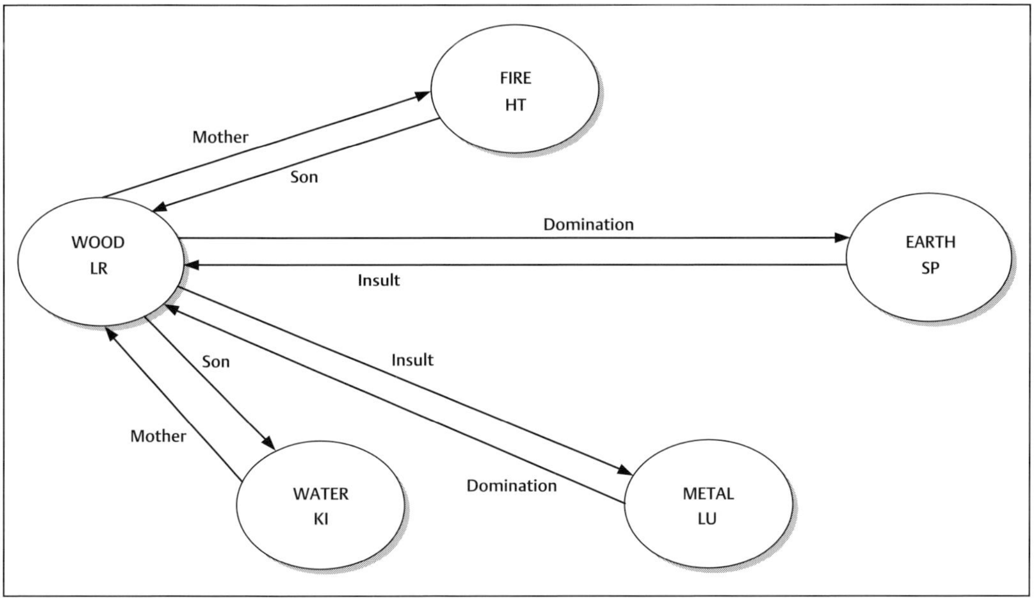

Figure 2–6 Wood complete movements.

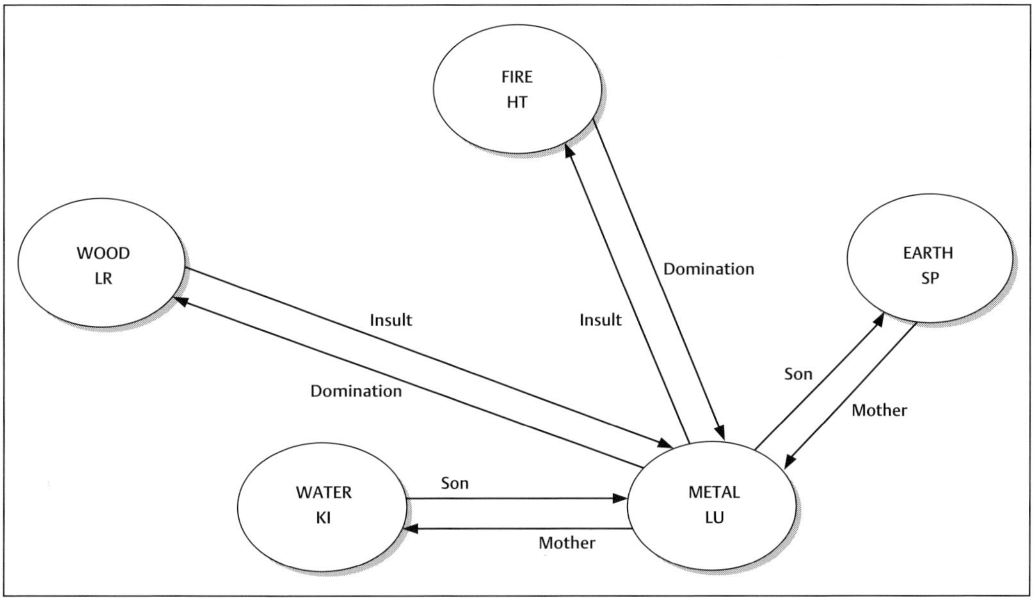

Figure 2–7 Metal complete movements.

ficult expectoration, and/or hyperthyroidism. When the kidneys (water) overact on the heart (fire), the kidney *yin* is vacuous and empty; heat then forms that can be transmitted to the heart and becomes a factor in panic, depression, and/or essential hypertension.

When the relationships among phases turn to a rebellion (*Wu*) cycle, pathological conditions will result. When the liver (wood) insults the lungs (metal), the liver *qi* can stagnate upward and obstruct the chest and breathing. When the heart (fire) insults the kidneys (water), the heart

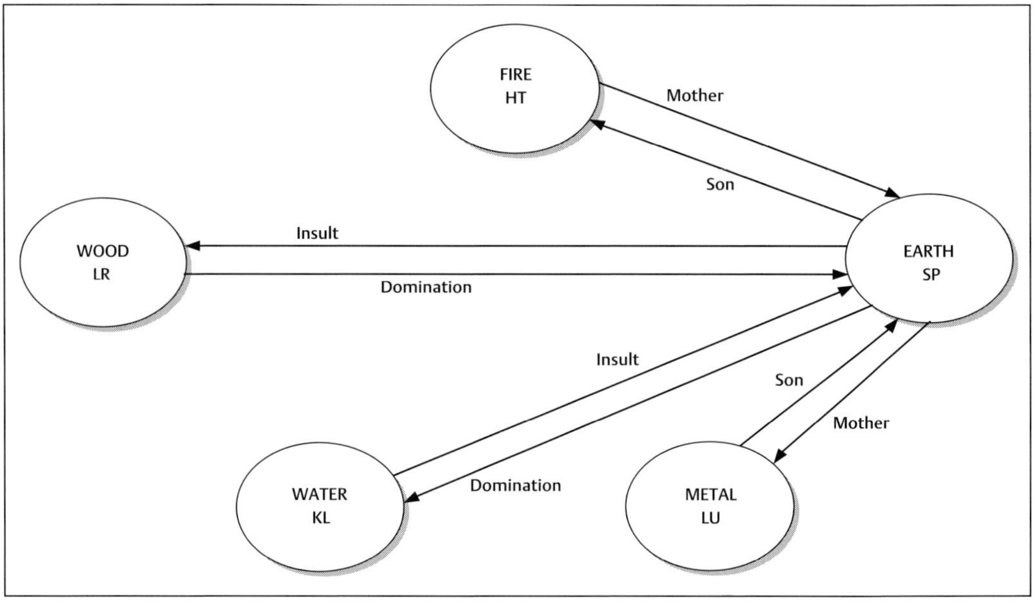

Figure 2–8 Earth complete movements.

fire can infuse downward into the kidneys and cause kidney *yin* vacuity and fatigue. When the spleen (earth) insults the liver (wood), the spleen retains dampness, which can impair the free flow of liver *qi*. When the lungs (metal) insult the heart (fire), the lungs are obstructed by phlegm and can impair the circulation of the heart *qi*. When the kidneys (water) insult the spleen (earth), the kidneys fail to transform fluids and the spleen and become obstructed by dampness.

If the engendering cycle goes awry, the mother phase is not nourishing the child phase or the child phase is taking too much from the mother phase. For example, if the liver (wood) 'mother' is affecting the heart (fire) 'child,' the liver fails to nourish the 'child' heart. When the liver blood is vacuous, it affects the heart blood, which becomes vacuous, and palpitations and insomnia will ensue. The gall bladder controls the capacity for decision making and courage. When the 'mother' gall bladder (wood) depletes itself for the child, it can affect the mind or heart (fire) causing emotional weakness, timidity, and lack of assertion. When the heart 'child' affects the liver 'mother,' heart blood is vacuous, which can affect the liver storage of blood, which could cause scanty periods or amenorrhea. When the heart 'mother' affects the spleen 'child,' the mind of the heart needs to support the mental faculties and the ability to concentrate, which belong to the spleen. When the heart 'fire' is vacuous, the spleen is unable to warm and a cold feeling in the body and diarrhea ensue. When the spleen 'child' affects the heart 'mother,' the spleen makes *qi* and blood but the heart needs a strong supply of blood. If there is not enough blood from the spleen, palpitations, insomnia, slight depression, and poor memory can occur. When the spleen 'mother' affects the lung 'child,' phlegm will be formed, which often settles in the lungs causing breathlessness and asthma. When the lung 'child' affects the spleen 'mother,' lung *qi* is vacuous and spleen *qi* will be affected causing tiredness, no appetite, and loose stools.

When the lung's 'mother' depletes itself for the 'child' kidney, the lung *qi* is vacuous. The *qi* in the fluids cannot descend to the kidneys, causing breathlessness. The kidney is unable to receive the *qi* and dryness of the kidneys ensues. When the kidney 'child' affects the lung 'mother,' *qi* will rebel upward and obstruct the lungs causing breathlessness. When the kidney 'mother' affects the liver 'child,' if the kidney *yin* is vacuous, the liver *yin* and blood will become vacuous giving rise to tinnitus, dizziness, headaches, and irritability. When the liver 'child' affects the kidney 'mother,' if the liver blood is vacuous over a long period of time, it can lead to vacuity of kidney essence causing dizziness, tinnitus, night sweats, and sexual weakness.

Therefore, each of the five phases can be out of balance in the following ways:

- The restraining (*Ke*) cycle direction becomes *replete* and *overacts* upon the controllee phase, becoming the overwhelming (*Cheng*) cycle.
- The restraining (*Ke*) cycle direction becomes *vacuous* and the *qi* flows in the opposite direction, *insulting* the controller phase becoming the rebellion (*Wu*) cycle.
- The engendering (*Sheng*) cycle becomes *replete* and draws excessively from the mother phase resulting in a weak mother.
- The engendering (*Sheng*) cycle becomes *vacuous* and fails to nourish the child, resulting in a weak child.

Traditional Chinese Medicine Philosophy of Pathology

Chinese medicine lists most illnesses as a disturbance in the flow of *qi*. This can be one of three possible states. The *qi*, or vital energy, may be replete, vacuous, or stagnant in the organ(s) or the channel(s).

Vacuous *qi* conditions are characterized by weakness of *qi* and inadequate function of organs; this is called the *xu* conditions. Typical illnesses that arise with a disturbance involving vacuity of *qi* are degenerative illnesses, diseases of old age, and mental depression. Cardinal symptoms occur as pallor, cold hands and feet, low blood pressure, lack of drive, and lack of energy.

Repletion *qi* conditions are referred to as *shi* or *yang* conditions. They include symptoms such as flushing, acute shooting or cramping pain, uneasiness, nervousness, and excitement.

The main symptom of *qi* stagnation is pain. The usual result of stagnation of *qi* is called *zhi zheng*. Symptoms include high muscle tone, muscle pain, myalgias, restricted movement, and headache. External causes of stagnation include climatic instances that lead to blockage of *qi* in the channels such as heat, cold, dryness, dampness, wind, or any combination. The internal causes of stagnation of *qi* include faulty nutrition, and mental or emotional stress. These mental/emotional states include fear, rage, anger, brooding, agitation, and sadness. Finally, other causes of disease leading to stagnation are overexcitation, excessive mental or physical work, accumulation of phlegm, infections, trauma, and excessive sexual or physical activity.[20]

Diagnosis by Eight Principles of Traditional Chinese Medicine

TCM uses diagnosis by the Eight Principles method, listed in **Figure 2–9**. The traditional system classifies the individual signs and symptoms of illness according to diametrically opposed diagnostic criteria. These eight diagnostic criteria are known as the *Ba gang*, which are interior/ exterior (*li biao*), vacuity/ repletion (*xu shi*), cold/ heat (*han re*), and *Yin*/*Yang*.[21]

Interior disturbances, called *li*, are states of the five *zang* organs and the six *fu* organs. They are frequently chronic in nature and are characterized by pains in the thoracic and abdominal area with symptoms such as nausea and diarrhea. They can also cause symptoms of fear, anxiety, and excitement.

External illnesses are called *biao*. They are characterized by disturbances in the channels and the collateral channels in the peripheral regions on the surface of the body. They typically include peripheral neuralgia and localized joint disease. Chinese medicine considered these causes external, climatic, and related to pathogenic influences such as cold, heat, damp, wind, or dryness.

Vacuity syndromes include vacuities of *qi*, blood, or *jing*. These typical symptoms are tiredness, exhaustion, dizziness, motor retardation, low blood pressure, inadequate blood perfusion and vacuity of body fluids. These vacuity conditions are usually chronic.

Interior	←→	Exterior
Cold	←→	Hot
Vacuous	←→	Replete
Yin	←→	*Yang*

Figure 2–9 Eight principles of Traditional Chinese Medicine.

Disturbances caused by repletion or *shi* are described as a repletion of *qi* or blood in the organs or channels. They include symptoms of acute pain, cramps, hypertension, increased muscle tone, and increased secretion of body fluids. Redness of the face, and a strong pulse are important physical signs. Patients may demonstrate nervousness, agitation, restlessness, and sleeplessness.

Cold disturbances, or *han*, occur when external pathogenic cold takes effect on the body. Cold disturbances are usually chronic and the symptoms include the feeling of coldness in the extremities and pallor.

Heat disturbances, *re*, are caused by increased *yang* activity of the *qi* within the body. Thus, *yin/yang* is used in the diagnosis. Overactivity of *yang* leads to exhaustion of *yin* forces and fluids. Therefore, if they persist, a *yang* heat may result. This includes high body temperature, redness, hyperthermia, pain, and agitation.[21]

The eight diagnostic criteria seldom occur in isolation but rather in combination. For example, repletion and heat often occur together. Repletion and cold can also occur simultaneously as well as vacuity and heat, see **Table 2–10**.

Table 2–10 Symptoms of heat and cold

Heat: *re*	**Cold: *han***
Red face	Pale face
Redness of skin	Pale skin
Red mucous menbranes	Pale mucous membranes
Warmness	Coolness
Burning of the extremities	Cold extremities
Fever	Hypothermia
Feeling hot	Feeling cold
Exacerbation of symptoms of heat	Exacerbation of symptoms of cold
Thirst for cold fluids	Need for warm drinks
Dark, scanty urine	Dilute urine
Constant constipation	Watery stool
Fast pulse	Slow pulse
Red tongue	Pale tongue

Chinese medicine describes pain in two different classifications: *xu*, which is vacuity, and *shi*, which is repletion, consult **Table 2–11**. *Shi* generally represents the most painful conditions due to stagnation of *qi* and/or blood, and stagnation due to cold. *Xu* pain can result from insufficient nourishment of *qi* and/or blood, which results in the retardation of the circulation of *qi* and blood.

In conclusion, the most common causative factors of pain according to TCM are:

- Stagnation of *qi*
- Stagnation of blood
- Accumulation of cold
- Accumulation of heat
- Retention of phlegm.

Table 2–11 Symptoms of repletion and vacuity

Repletion: *shi*	**Vacuity: *xu***
Acute pain	Dull pain
Powerful muscular movements	Febrile, slow muscular movements
Agitation	Tiredness
Hyperactivity	Exhaustion
Loud voice	Faint voice
Upright posture	Stooped posture
Quick gait	Slow gait
Hypertension	Hypotension
Hyperemia	Vacuous blood perfusion
Psychologically active attitude	Psychological passivity
Excitement, mania	Depression
Replete activity	Subdued mood; vacuous activity
Short sleep period	Long sleep period
Coated tongue	Little tongue coating
Strong pulse	Weak pulse

Acupuncture Channel Theory

Jing luo is the Chinese description for the system of channels and their collaterals. *Jing* are the channels. The original meaning of the ideogram *jing* is the warp threads in weaving. The longitudinal threads provide the structure of the woven fabric, as the channels are the structural phases of the body. *Luo* means to connect, to knot. The *luo* vessels connect the coupled or paired channels with each other.[22]

Acupuncture channels and connecting vessels are pathways that allow *qi*, blood, and body fluids (moisture) to move throughout the body. *The Canon of Perplexities* states, "The channels move blood and *qi* and ensure the free flow of *yin* and *yang*, so that the body is properly nourished."[23] There are two major channels—the organ-related regular channels and the eight extraordinary vessels or curious channels. "There are regular channels and extraordinary vessels. The 12 channels are the regular channels. The Eight Extraordinary vessels are so named because they do not conform to the norm. *Qi* and blood constantly flow through the 12 regular channels and when abundant overflow into the extraordinary vessels."[23] For the eight extraordinary vessels, see **Table 2–12**.

Channel theory is important in that, physiologically, these 12 channels represent the principal pathways by which *qi*, blood, and moisture are distributed around the body providing nourishment and health. Here is how the *Ling Shu* describes the channels: "the channels are the routes by which blood and *qi* move and *yin* and *yang* circulate, keeping the bones and sinews moistened and the joints lubricated."[23]

Table 2–12 The eight extraordinary vessels

	Master point	Coupled point
Ren mai	LU-7	KI-6
Du mai	SI-3	BL-26
Chong mai	SP-4	PC-6
Dai mai	GB-41	TB-5
Yin qiao	KI-6	LU-7
Yang qiao	BL-62	SI-3
Yin wei	PC-6	SP-4
Yang wei	TB-5	GB-41

Qi is the activating force for the movement of blood and moisture in the channels. Exogenous pathogens invade the body's defensive *qi* through the exterior and penetrate the interior of the body through the channels, thereby affecting the corresponding organs.

The 12 channels are bilaterally symmetrical. They are identified according to the limb they flow on, the organ they are associated with, and *yin* or *yang*, according to their nature. *Yin* channels are on the anterior and medial surfaces of the trunk and inner surfaces of the limbs. *Yang* channels are on the posterior and lateral surfaces of the trunk and the outer surfaces of the limb. The 11 organs in Chinese medicine intersect intimately with the channels. These organs are more functional systems in Chinese medicine; for example, the lung channel is anatomically correlated from nasal passages to bronchial tubes, as opposed to solely the lung parenchyma.

There are five *yang* organs called *fu* organs. These are hollow organs and their functions are similar to those described in Western medicine. They are the small intestine, gall bladder, large intestine, stomach, and bladder; with the triple burner, a channel without an organ. There are six *yin* organs called *zang* organs. They are the heart, liver, lung, spleen, kidney, and pericardium. *Yang* channels are related to hollow viscera (organs) and *yin* channels are related to solid viscera (organs).[23] The interior–exterior relationship of the 12 regular, *zang fu*, channels has two components, see **Table 2–2**:

- Each *yang* (*fu*) Hollow organ connects with one *yin* (*zang*) solid organ.
- Each solid organ *yin* (*zang*) connects with its corresponding *yang* (*fu*) hollow organ.

Each channel communicates up and down the body through a related hand and foot channel. They communicate with each other as the *qi*, blood, and moisture move through the channels as shown in **Table 2–13**. The flow of *qi* is constant but there is a regular sequenced cycle through the channels every 24 hours (**Table 2–4**).

Table 2–13 Twelve channels of *qi* table

Fu Channel	Limb	*Yin/Yang* Identity	Pathway	Related *Zang* Channel to Which *Qi* Flows
LU	Hand	*Tai yin*	Anterior portion of the inside of the arm	LI
SP	Foot	*Tai yin*	Anterior portion of the inside of the leg	HT
LI	Hand	*Yang ming*	Anterior portion of the outside of the arm	ST
ST	Foot	*Yang ming*	Anterior portion of the outside of the leg	SP
HT	Hand	*Shao yin*	Posterior portion of the inside of the arm	SI
KI	Foot	*Shao yin*	Posterior portion of the inside of the leg	HT
SI	Hand	*Tai yang*	Posterior portion of the outside of the arm	BL
BL	Foot	*Tai yang*	Posterior portion of the outside of the leg	KI
PC	Hand	*Jue yin*	Middle portion of the inside of the arm	TB
LR	Foot	*Jue yin*	Middle portion of the inside of the leg	PC
TB	Hand	*Shao yang*	Middle portion of the outside of the arm	GB
GB	Foot	*Shao yang*	Middle portion of the outside of the leg	LR

Acupuncture Channel Distribution

Acupuncture channels traverse throughout the entire body through the various regions of the body. Different channels are on the skin surface at different parts of the body. This distribution of channels has important theoretical and practical relationships to the body.

Of the 12 regular channels and eight extraordinary channels, there are a total of eight channels that circulate up to the head. These are the governing vessel, bladder, triple burner, gall bladder, liver, stomach, *yang wei*, and *yang qiao*.

The following is a description of channels that pass through the head. The governing vessel arises from the lower abdomen and emerges from the perineum, it then runs posterior along the interior spinal column to the nape of the neck where it enters the brain and ascends to the vertex of the head and winds along the forehead to the columella of the nose.

The bladder channel starts from the inner canthus, ascends to the forehead, and joins the governing vessel at the vertex where a branch arises, running to the temple. A straight portion of the channel enters and communicates with the brain from the vertex of the head and emerges and bifurcates to descend along the posterior aspect of the neck. It then moves down to the lumbar region connecting to the kidney and joining the bladder. It then travels down to the outside of the tuberosity of the fifth metatarsal bone and reaches the lateral aspect of the tip of the little toe.

The gall bladder channel originates in the outer canthus, ascends to the corner of the forehead, and curves downward to the retroauricular region. It then runs along the side of the neck in front of the triple burner to the shoulder down to the supraclavicular fossa where it further descends into the chest through the diaphragm, entering the gall bladder, and down the lateral side of the abdomen/hip region, going further down along the anterior aspect of the tibia. Finally, it reaches the anterior aspect of the external malleolus, then to the dorsum of the foot on the lateral side of the tip of the fourth toe.

The liver channel starts from the dorsum of the great toe running upward along the dorsum of the foot in front of the medial malleolus. It then moves up the medial side of the knee and curves around the external genitalia and comes up the lower abdomen through the diaphragm, ascending to the posterior aspect of the throat. From the throat to the nasal pharynx, the liver channel connects with the ocular system. Continuing upward, it emerges from the forehead and meets the governing vessel at the vertex of the head. A branch arises from the ocular region and runs downward into the cheek and curves around the inner surface of the lips.

The stomach channel starts in the lateral side of the ala nasi and ascends to the bridge of the nose where it meets the bladder channel turning downward along the lateral side of the nose. It enters the upper gums and curves around the lips, descending to meet the conception vessel, *ren mai*, at the mentolabial groove. It then runs posteriorly laterally across the lower portion of the cheek, winding along the angle of the mandible, ascending in front of the ear, and traverses the gall bladder channel, where it follows the anterior hairline and reaches the forehead. The facial branch emerging from ST-5, *da ying*, runs down toward ST-9, *ren ying*, from there it goes along the throat and enters the supraclavicular fossa, descending through the diaphragm and entering the stomach to connect with the spleen. The stomach channel runs downward passing through the nipple and descends past the umbilicus bilaterally to the lower abdomen. It continues running caudally, reaching the knee; from there it continues downward along the anterior border of the lateral aspect of the tibia and follows the dorsum of the foot to the lateral side of the tip of the second toe.

The triple burner originates in the tip of the ring finger moving upward to the dorsal aspect of the wrist and the lateral aspect of the forearm and lateral aspect of the upper arm. It reaches the shoulder region where it passes behind the gall bladder channel, winding over the supraclavicular fossa, spreading into the chest to connect with the pericardium. It then descends through the diaphragm down to the abdomen and joins the upper, middle, and lower burners, *jiao*. A branch from the chest runs upward, emerges from the supraclavicular fossa, and further descends to the neck, running along the posterior border of the ear to the corner of the anterior hairline. It then turns toward the cheek and terminates in the infraorbital region. The auricular branch arises from the retroauricular region and enters the ear. This branch then emerges in front of the ear crossing the previous branch of the cheek and reaches the outer canthus.

The extraordinary channel, *yang wei*, originates in the foot at BL-63 (*jin men*). It emerges from the external malleolus, ascends along the gall bladder channel through the hip region running upward along the hypochondrial regions to the posterior aspect of the shoulder. It then moves backward to the back of the neck where it communicates with the governing vessel, *du mai*.

The extraordinary channel, *yang qiao*, starts from the lateral surface of the heel at BL-61 (*pu can*). It runs upward along the external malleolus and passes the posterior border of the fibula, moving along the lateral surface of the thigh to the posterior axillary fold. From there, it winds over the shoulder and ascends along the neck to the corner of the mouth. It enters the intercanthus at BL-1 (*jing ming*) and communicates with the *yin qiao* channel, running further upward along the bladder channel to the forehead, meeting the gall bladder channel at GB-20 (*feng chi*).[24]

The following is a description of the channels by area of the head.

Vertex

The bladder channel intersects with the vertex of the head while the governing vessel, *du mai*, crosses the vertex. The liver channel meets the governing vessel near the vertex with the triple burner channel branches and moves toward the vertex. The gall bladder channel traverses at the vertex of the scalp. The governing vessel belongs to the brain, whereas the bladder channel connects with the brain.

The stomach channel branch passes through the eyes and enters the brain. In the forehead, the stomach channel follows the anterior hairline to the center of the forehead. The bladder channel rises up across the forehead. The liver channel runs up the forehead. The gall bladder channel rises to the lateral corners of the forehead. The triple burner channel finishes at the lateral corner of the forehead. The kidney, spleen, stomach, heart, and small intestine channels all have connecting vessels that meet in the ear and rise to connect to the lateral corners of the forehead.

Face

The head is the confluence of *yang*. All *yang* channels pass through the head. The liver channel travels through the nose and throat eventually reaching the vertex. The conception and governing vessels, *ren mai* and *du mai*, traverse the face, while the gall bladder channel divergence disappears, moving laterally away from the face.

The liver opens at the eyes. The liver, heart, stomach, and gall bladder channels all go to the eyes. The *yin* and *yang* motility vessels reach the canthus. The gall bladder, bladder, small intestine, and triple burner channels all approach the eye. The bladder channel traverses the upper eyelid, the stomach channel begins below the lower eyelid. The lung opens the nose and the stomach channel connects at the nose as well as at the bladder. The large intestine, stomach, and small intestine channels all traverse the nasal region. The liver channel reaches the nasopharyngeal cavity. In the suborbital and paranasal regions, the bladder and stomach channels meet at the side of the nose. The stomach channel traverses the suborbital region. The large intestine channel terminates at the side of the nose. The small intestine channel branches into the suborbital region. The triple burner channel goes into the suborbital region. The gall bladder channel passes through the suborbital region. The stomach channel divergence rises to the suborbital region.

Mouth

The conception vessel (*ren mai*) traverses the submandibular region. The stomach channel flows along the lower angle of the mandible. The triple burner channel divergence begins in the submandibular region. The gall bladder channel travels to the submandibular region and meets the small intestine channel at the submandibular region. The triple burner rises to the submandibular region. The large intestine channel passes through the submandibular region. The lower angle of the jaw has the gall bladder and stomach channel traversing through it. The lips and mouth have the stomach channel skirting along the upper and lower lips. The liver channel contours the inside of the lip.The large intestine channel pinches the mouth from both sides. The stomach channel divergence begins at the mouth.

A branch of the large intestine connecting vessel spreads over the teeth, and the stomach channel enters the upper teeth. The large intestine channel spreads through the lower teeth.

The heart channel opens the tongue. The triple burner channel connects with the root of the tongue. The bladder channel branches into and meets at the root of the tongue. The spleen channel disperses over the inferior surface of the tongue. The kidney channel divergence connects to the root of the tongue.

Ear

The ear has many channels that traverse and connect to it. The bladder channel goes to the apex of the ear, and the gall bladder channel descends behind the ear, enters the ear, and travels anteriorly. The stomach channel rises in front of the ear. The small intestine channel enters the ear. The triple burner channel goes behind the ear and comes out at the apex of the ear; it also enters the ear and travels anteriorly. The large intestine channel connecting vessel enters into the ear. The gall bladder channel also follows behind the ear. The stomach channel meets anterior to the ear. The small intestine channel meets behind the ear and a branch enters the ear and goes to the apex. The pericardium divergence begins behind the ear and unites with the triple burner divergence. The connecting vessels of the kidney, heart, lungs, and stomach all meet at the ear. In the occiput of the head, the bladder channel and governing vessel traverse. The gall bladder channel traverses the parietal and occipital regions along with the bladder channels medially.

Scientific Physiological Effects of Acupuncture

Acupuncture analgesia for humans has been reported for thousands of years in China and it has been explained and reported in veterinary medicine over the past 1000 years in China and for the past 100 years in Europe.[25] The basic questions of acupuncture analgesia are: Does it really work? And if it works, what is the scientific mechanism?

Since 1973, hundreds of research papers have been written regarding the clinical effectiveness of acupuncture.[25] The neurological mechanism of acupuncture analgesia starts with the hypothesis that "acupuncture analgesia is initiated by small diameter nerves in muscles which send impulses to the spinal cord and then to the three centers: spinal column, midbrain, and pituitary are activated to release transmitter chemicals (endorphins and monoamines) to block the 'pain' messages."[25] The small diameter myelinated and unmyelinated nerve types II, III, IV, A, and C carry pain messages. Types IV and C are unmyelinated, and types II, III, and A are myelinated. The large diameter myelinated nerves A-Beta and type I, carry touch or proprioception, respectively. Pain from an injury starts at the skin that activates the sensory receptors of the small afferent nerve fibers of A-delta and C-axon size. This afferent pain is carried to the spinothalamic tract in the spinal cord and projects its axon to the thalamus to ultimately synapse into the cortex to activate the primary somatosensory area.[25]

When an acupuncture needle is placed in the skin and muscle, a sensory receptor sends an impulse to the spinal cord to type II and III muscle afferent nerves. Type II small diameter myelinated afferents are thought to signal the numbness of *de qi* needling sensation and type III provides the mild aching sensation of the acupuncture. The unmyelinated type IV afferent nerves from the muscle provide the soreness that is felt when the acupuncture needle is placed. Biochemical stimulation from the acupuncture needle is through the afferent nerves synapse in the spinal cord onto the anterolateral tract, which projects into the spinal cord, midbrain, and pituitary hypothalamic cortex. It is within the spinal cord that the endorphinergic cell releases either enkephalin or dynorphin. The spinal cord endorphins, particularly β-endorphin, cause a presynaptic inhibition of the painful message. Thus, enkephalin and dynorphin block pain transmission at the spinal cord level. The presynaptic inhibition probably works by reducing calcium inflow during the change of action potential in the membrane.[25]

Acupuncture stimulation of nerve fibers in the muscles sending impulses to the spinal cord, midbrain, and pituitary hypothalamic cortex causes analgesia. "The spinal site uses enkephalin and dynorphin to block incoming messages at low frequency and other transmitters such as gamma-aminobutyric acid (GABA) with the electrical stimulation at high frequency. The midbrain uses enkephalin to activate the raphe descending system which inhibits spinal cord pain transmission by a synergistic effect by the monoamines, serotonin, and norepinephrine. The midbrain also has a circuit which bypasses the endorphinergic links at high frequency stimulation. At the third center, the hypothalamus pituitary, the pituitary releases beta-enkephalin into the blood and cerebral spinal fluid to cause analgesia at a distance. The hypothalamus also sends long axons to the midbrain and by beta-endorphins it activates the descending analgesia system. This third center is activated not at high frequency but at low frequency stimulation."[25]

Low frequency is defined as 2 to 4 Hz. High frequency is defined as 50 to 200 Hz. The high frequency, low intensity needling bypasses the endorphin system, whereas the low frequency, high intensity needling works through the endorphin system and acts on all three centers.

The evidence of how acupuncture works has been demonstrated through thousands of research articles published in both Asia and the West. One particular researcher, Bruce Pomeranz, lists 17 different lines of experimental scientific evidence in his book, *Basics of Acupuncture*, with Gabriel Stux, to prove the neural humural and physiological effects of acupuncture. They are:

1. Many different opiate antagonists block acupuncture analgesia.
2. Naloxone has a stereo-specific effect.
3. Microinjection of naloxone blocks acupuncture analgesia only if given into analgesic sites in the central nervous system.
4. Mice genetically vacuous in opiate receptors show poor acupuncture analgesia.
5. Rats vacuous in endorphin show poor anesthesia.
6. Endorphin levels in blood and cerebral spinal fluid fall in specific brain regions during acupuncture analgesia.
7. Acupuncture analgesia is enhanced by protecting endorphins from enzyme degradation.
8. Acupuncture analgesia can be transmitted to a second animal by cerebral spinal fluid transfer or by cross–circulation, and its effect is blocked by naloxone.
9. Reduction of pituitary endorphins suppresses acupuncture analgesia.

10. There is a rise in mRNA for proenkephalin in brain and pituitary lasting 24 to 48 hours after 30 minutes of electrical acupuncture, indicating a prolonged increased level of enkephalin, which could explain the enduring effects of electrical acupuncture and the potentiation of repeated daily treatments.
11. There is a cross-tolerance between acupuncture analgesia and morphine analgesia implicating endorphins in acupuncture analgesia.
12. Acupuncture analgesia is more effective against emotional aspects of pain compared to pharmacological methods alone.
13. Lesions of the arcuate nucleus of the hypothalamus abolish acupuncture analgesia.
14. Lesions of the periaquaductal gray in the midbrain abolish acupuncture analgesia.
15. The level of C-FOS gene protein is elevated in endorphin-related areas of the brain during acupuncture analgesia.
16. The addition of monoamines mediates the effects of 100 hz electrical acupuncture, dynorphine may also be involved; thus at 100 hz there is an elevation of dynorphin levels in the dorsal horn of rats' spinal cords. In lumbar punctures in humans receiving 100 hz electrical acupuncture, there is an elevation of dynorphin A. Rats given electrical acupuncture at 100 hz showed acupuncture analgesia, which is blocked by the dynorphin kappa antagonists, while the electrical acupuncture at 2 hz is blocked by mu and delta antagonists, suggesting the involvement of enkephalins and β-endorphins at these low frequencies.
17. Electrical acupuncture in rats elevated precursors of the three endorphins: proenkephalin, preprodynorphine, and preproendorphin mRNA.[26]

Several experiments involving the pituitary gland were performed, both surgical removal of the pituitary and suppression of the pituitary endorphins by chemical manipulations. All of these experiments suppressed acupuncture analgesia in animals. Another experiment involved spinal cord blockage of serotonin receptors and blockage of serotonin synthesis by direct microinjection of naloxone into the midbrain. The midbrain showed that morphine pain relief was largely mediated by this system. Experiments included direct lesions to the median rafe by cutting the output fibers in the dorsal lateral tract. All of these experiments reduced acupuncture analgesia. Enhancement of serotonin synthesis increases acupuncture analgesia; an acupuncture experiment measuring serotonin showed increased production occurred during acupuncture analgesia along with noradrenaline affecting the release of endorphins verify and support the mechanisms of acupuncture analgesia.[27]

Acupuncture does not work 100% of the time. Individuals with elevated cholecystikinin (CCK) in the central nervous system are poor responders to acupuncture analgesia because CCK has been shown to block the acupuncture effect by acting on the periaqueductal gray matter. 25 Acupuncture has been shown not to be physiologically addicting, but acupuncture has been shown to be additive and cumulative, with its effect becoming more powerful after 10 to 15 treatments.[28]

In conclusion, acupuncture works neurologically by stimulating the small myelinated A-delta type III fibers and it does not work on the large C fibers. There is now a large body of scientific evidence that indicates there are several causes and effects of acupuncture. Acupuncture has been shown to be effective for both acute and chronic pain conditions. It has been found to be effective for the treatment of addiction and withdrawal from various drugs, diseases of the gastrointestinal, environmental, cardiovascular, neurological, and immunological systems. The World Health Organization (WHO) has been very active in the determination of the usefulness and indications for acupuncture worldwide. 29 They have determined acupuncture to be effective in treatment of the disorders and illnesses listed in **Table 2–14**.

Theories Regarding YNSA

The description of traditional Chinese medicine acupuncture theory, its origins, and recent scientific investigations of how and why acupuncture works was presented. To understand the uniqueness of YSNA scalp acupuncture, one needs to start from what is known to go further into the unknown as one pursues the development of YNSA. Starting with the knowledge of anatomy, physiology, pathology, acupuncture traditions,

Table 2–14 Indications for acupuncture treatment as primary or complementary[30]

Respiratory tract disorders	**Neurological and orthopedic disorders (cont.)**
– Acute sinusitis	– Bell's palsy
– Acute rhinitis	– Causalgia
– Acute tonsillitis	– Cervicalgia
– Common cold	– Classical and common migraine
Bronchopulmonary disorders	– CVA
– Acute and chronic bronchitis	– Depression
– Bronchial asthma	– Dysarthria
– Upper respiratory tract infections	– Entrapment neuropathy
Disorders of the eye	– Facial paralysis
– Acute conjunctivitis	– Headache
– Central rhinitis	– Hearing loss
– Cataract without complications	– Hemiplegia
– Myopia (in children)	– Herniated cervical disc
Disorders of the oral cavity	– Herniated lumbar disc
– Acute and chronic pharyngitis	– Intercostal neuralgia
– Gingivitis	– Lateral epicondylitis
– Pain after tooth extraction	– Lower motor neuron disease
– TMJ dysfunction	– Lumbago
– Toothache	– Mechanical low back pain
Endocrine system disorders	– Medial epicondylitis
– Diabetes mellitus type II	– Menière's disease
– Hyperthyroidism	– Migraine
– Hypothyroidism	– Myelitis
Gastrointestinal disorders	– Neurogenic bladder dysfunction
– Acute and chronic colitis	– Osteoarthritis
– Acute and chronic gastritis	– Nocturnal enuresis
– Acute bacterial dysentery	– Paralysis after apoplectic fit
– Chronic duodenal ulcer	– Paralysis caused by poliomyelitis
– Constipation	– Paraplegia
– Crohn's disease	– Periarthritis humeroscapularis
– Diarrhea	– Peripheral neuropathy
– Dysphasia	– Reflex sympathetic dystrophy
– Gastric hyperacidity	– Rheumatoid arthritis
– Gastroptosis	– Sciatica
– Hiccoughs	– Somatic dysfunction of the head, cervical spine, thoracic spine, lumbar spine, sacrum, pelvis, lower extremity, upper extremity, rib cage, or abdomen
– Paralytic ileus	– Tennis elbow
– Spasm of the esophagus	– Tension headache
Genital/urinary system disorders	– Tinnitus
– Renal pain	– Transient ischemic attack
– Urinary tract infection	– Trigeminal neuralgia
Neurological and orthopedic disorders	– Upper motor neuron disease
– Anxiety	
– Aphasia: Broca's and Wernicke's	
– Asnomia	

CVA, cerebrovascular accident; TMJ, temporomandibular joint.

and systems, one is able to move from tradition to science.

The scientific research regarding acupuncture's effect is assumed to be the same for YNSA as it is for TCM. In essence, YNSA places a needle on the scalp, which affects the central nervous system, resulting in observed broad and often distant effects. The placement of the needle over a YNSA acupoint is always, with rare exception, a small palpatory hill or mountain of the subcutaneous scalp tissue. This YNSA acupoint is not usually over a traditional Chinese acupuncture channel point. Though the needle is placed in a nontraditional acupuncture point, one can assume because of the rich plexi of neural, arterial, and venule plexi that the same and similar neural effects take place as discussed by the 17 lines of scientific acupuncture research introduced by Stux and Pomeranz earlier in this chapter. If one accepts the scientific truth of acupuncture and acupuncture's demonstrated effects upon the entire body, then what are the reason(s) for one specific scalp point having such a dramatic effect? To answer that question, one needs to investigate the quantum physics that are directly related to YNSA. One explanation is the Fractal Field Model, a theoretical model developed by Mandelbrot.[31]

Fractal Field Theory

According to the principle of fractalization, an organism creates many quantum copies of itself with projections onto the skin and mucous membranes. The biological reason for these multiple copies is to create a bigger, durable reserve for the informational structure and the development of the organism in time and space.

Benoit Mandelbrot was a scientist working in the field of nonlinear equations and complex numbers; he is the father of fractal geometry. Mandlebrot's set, Xn+1 = Xn2 + C, provides particular parameters that can be represented pictorially via computer graphics. A graphic display illustrates the variety of forms that arise coupled with self-similarity of the figures. This selfsimilarity is independent of size or scale.

In essence, the primary, or mother figure, gives rise to the smaller figures, which are still similar in form and content. This self-similarity is mathematically endless in principle, all the way down to the size of an atom. Apart from the principle of self-organization, one can see the dialectical unity of order and chaos within the same process.[31]

This fractalization principle has been recognized as a basic principle of nature in its self-organization and replication. One of the modern views regarding the explanation for the nature of acupuncture channels is the use of the Fractal Field Model. This is a way to describe the channels as a wave's extreme cycle in the organism's coherent field with projection onto the body surface at the acupuncture points. According to the positions, the main functions of the channels are an information exchange between the organism and the environment.[32] Fractal electromagnetic fields are able to transmit information without energy transfer and are dependent on the role of material substratum, by means of which the exchange is realized.[33]

The advantage to a physician in using a microsystem, such as YNSA, is that the main task is to find the core pathology, then find a proper portal to influence the organism through a single or multiple mechanism(s) directly or indirectly, with the goal being to bring about health and homeostasis within the physiological parameters of that human body. Sometimes it is much easier to do so using the microsystem where all the information about an individual is concentrated on a limited representative surface. The Fractal Field Model applied to a scalp microsystem of acupuncture provides a theoretical working process based on mathematics and physics. The YNSA methodology provides an easily usable clinical method of treating the whole person through just a few needles in one microsystem.

In summary, YNSA microsystem acupuncture is explained as one of the manifestations of fractalization (Fractal Field Model), the universal principle of self-organization within nature. The resolution of YNSA in its influence on the organism is dependent on the size of the projection of the organ on the scalp skin surface.[31]

Calcification Theory

It is the author's contention that because YNSA is biomechanically, physically separating the loose subcutaneous tissue of the scalp with the needle, particularly over the YNSA 'lines' (A-1–8, E-1–12, D-1–6, C-1,2) the resultant change in electrical conductivity occurs in the scalp. This electrical potential change affects the entire fascial system, including the periosteal membranes and dura mater. The biomechanical change is caused by both the biomechanics and the electrical potential of the needle placed in the scalp. With the needle placement, the electrical resistance of the skin is changed. The needle's bioelectrical potential and skin resistance interchange alters the biochemistry of the superficial and deep fascia of the scalp. This is discussed in more detail in Chapter 9. The calcium bridges that tightly bind the deep sheath of fascia to the periosteum cause an increase in electrical resistance. This electrical resistance may contribute to a deleterious effect on the patient's health. It is the author's theory that it is the mechanical breaking up of the microcalcium bridges with the YNSA needle that stimulates bioelectrical harmony and ultimately delivers a positive move toward health in the patient.

The YNSA needle's effect can be far-reaching. The needle's effect on the fascial chain linkage to the dura mater is quite probably based on the contiguous relationship from superficial to deep fascia, from deep fascia to periosteum, and from periosteum to dura mater. This calcium bridge affects the biochemistry and bioelectrical potentials of the organ and its metabolic processes. This biological activity change of the superficial scalp and the periosteum modifies the nervous system itself. This biomechanical → bioelectrical → biochemical change is transferred from the fascia to the biochemical changes within the brain—cerebrum, cerebellum, and brain stem first—then to the targeted organ through the nervous and circulatory systems, thereby effecting changes within the 12 channels. This bioelectrical change is clinically verified by a change in the Five Phase and TCM pulse diagnosis as well as with the YNSA neck and abdominal diagnosis findings after needle placement.[23]

Summary

Chinese medicine philosophy and terminology of *qi*, *yin* and *yang*, 12 channels, 8 extraordinary channels, *zang fu* organs, Eight Principles, and Five Phases are defined and discussed. The broad YNSA theory is that bodily functions can be affected and modified by placing acupuncture needles at very specific locations on the scalp to affect distant organs, acupuncture channels, and symptoms. It is similar to other microsystems in utilizing a small body region to affect the whole person, as explained by the Fractal Field Theory. One may only use YNSA Neck/Abdominal Diagnosis methods and treat using YNSA Basic and/or Ypsilon points, or one may use Five Phase or TCM diagnostic methods and pulse diagnosis to arrive at the same YNSA acupoints. However, to determine sidedness, as well as which quadrant to treat, YNSA Neck Diagnosis is required.

YNSA works because of quantum physics, Fractal Field Theory, the proven neurohumoral effects of body acupuncture, the electromagnetic effects of the acupuncture needle in the skin, and the biomechanical separation of high-density, electrical resistance microcalcium bridges on the scalp. Taken together, these factors cause biomechanical, biochemical, and bioelectrical changes resulting in subtle yet dramatic physiological and psychological changes in human health.

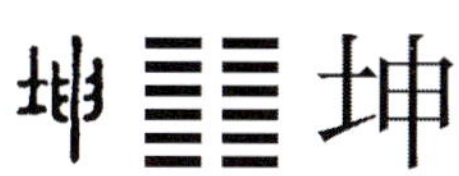

Kūn

Responding—Earth Above, Earth Below

*"*Yin *is the most gentle and submissive; when put in motion, it is strong and firm. Yin is the most quiet and still; when taking action, it is able to reach a definite goal."*[34]

"After heaven and earth have come into existence, myriad beings are produced. Qian and Kun are the origin, the source of Creation."[35]

References

Additional references are available on page 148.

1. Unschuld PU. Medicine in China: A History of Ideas. Berkeley: University of California Press; 1985: 277
2. Zheng-cai L, et al. A Study of Daoist Acupuncture and Moxibustion. Boulder, CO: Blue Poppy Press; 1999: 39–40
3. Kaptchuk TJ. The Web That Has No Weaver: Understanding Chinese Medicine. New York: McGraw-Hill; 1983: 3–4
4. Kendall DE. Problems with the Energy-Channel Theory. 2001. Available at: http://www.pacificcollege. edu/alumni/newsletters/summer2001/energy_ channel.html. Accessed January 8, 2005
5. Bensky D, O'Connor J. Acupuncture: A Comprehensive Text. Chicago: Eastland Press; 1981: 8
6. Stux G, Pomeranz B. Basics of Acupuncture. 5th ed. Berlin, Germany: Springer; 1998: 311
7. Garbacz E, Marshall S. Classical Chinese medicine: the science of biological forces. Medical Acupuncture 2000;12: 4
8. Mann F. Acupuncture: The Ancient Chinese Art of Healing and How It Works Scientifically. New York: First Vintage Books; 1973;47
9. Maciocia G. Foundations of Chinese Medicine: A Comprehensive Text for Acupuncturists and Herbalists. Edinburgh: Churchill Livingstone; 1989
10. Mann F. Acupuncture: The Ancient Chinese Art of Healing and How It Works Scientifically. New York: First Vintage Books; 1973;48
11. Stux G, Pomeranz B. Basics of Acupuncture. 5th ed. Berlin, Germany: Springer; 1998: 312
12. Matsumoto K, Birch S. Five Elements and Ten Stems: Nan Ching Theory, Diagnostics and Practice. New York: Paradigm Publications; 1983: 9–10
13. Bensky D, O'Connor J. Acupuncture: A Comprehensive Text. Chicago: Eastland Press; 1981: 10
14. Stux G, Pomeranz B. Basics of Acupuncture. 5th ed. Berlin, Germany: Springer; 1998: 310
15. Mann F. Acupuncture: The Ancient Chinese Art of Healing and How It Works Scientifically. New York: First Vintage Books; 1973: 61–62
16. Granet M. La Pensee Chinese [French]. Paris: Alban Michel. 1968: 367
17. Worsley JR. Classical Five-Element Acupuncture: The Five Elements and the Officials. New York: Redwing Book Co.; 1998: 1.1
18. Matsumoto K, Birch S. Five Elements and Ten Stems: Nan Ching Theory, Diagnostics and Practice. New York: Paradigm Publications; 1983: 13
19. Worsley JR. Classical Five-Element Acupuncture: The Five Elements and the Officials. New York: Redwing Book Co., 1998;3: 1.1–6.8
20. Stux G, Pomeranz B. Basics of Acupuncture. 5th ed. Berlin, Germany: Springer; 1998: 76
21. Stux G, Pomeranz B. Basics of Acupuncture. 5th ed. Berlin, Germany: Springer; 1998: 79–83
22. Stux G, Pomeranz B. Basics of Acupuncture. 5th ed. Berlin, Germany: Springer; 1998: 313
23. Ellis A, Wiseman N, Boss K. Fundamentals of Chinese Acupuncture. New York. Paradigm Publications 1991;29–31: 69
24. Mingqing Z. Zhu's Scalp Acupuncture. Hong Kong: Eight Dragons Publishing; 1992: 19–34
25. Stux G, Pomeranz B. Basics of Acupuncture. 5th ed. Berlin, Germany: Springer; 1998: 6–10, 12
26. Stux G, Pomeranz B. Basics of Acupuncture. 5th ed. Berlin, Germany: Springer; 1998: 17–18
27. Stux G, Pomeranz B. Basics of Acupuncture. 5th ed. Berlin, Germany: Springer; 1998: 15–23
28. Stux G, Pomeranz B. Basics of Acupuncture. 5th ed. Berlin, Germany: Springer; 1998: 13
29. Stux G, Pomeranz B. Basics of Acupuncture. 5th ed. Berlin, Germany: Springer; 1998: 307
30. Bannerman RH. Akupunktur: Die Ansicht der WHO. Weltgesundheit-Magazin der WHO. 1979: 12
31. Bouevitch V. Microacupuncture systems as fractals of the human body. The Web-Journal of Acupuncture. 1996. Available at:http://users.med.auth.gr/~karanik/ english/articles/micros.html. Accessed January 29, 2004
32. Nebrat V. The physical model of the low energy electromagnetic field influence on the human body through acupuncture points. Acupuncture White Nights '97. Saint-Petersburg: 2nd European Congress; 1997. Poster
33. Shipov G. The Physical Vacuum Theory. Moscow: NT-Center; 1993: 362
34. Huang A. The Complete I Ching. Rochester, VT: Inner Traditions; 1998: 43
35. Huang A. The Complete I Ching. Rochester, VT: Inner Traditions; 1998: 22

3

Energy and Healing in YNSA

"In every culture and in every medical tradition before ours, healing was accomplished by moving energy"[17] *– Albert Szent-Györgyi*

Energy Medicine History

Energy fields have been identified and used in medical context from more than 2500 years before the birth of Christ, when sick people were exposed to the shocks produced by electric eels. At different times, in different cultures, various stones/minerals were used in healing, from iron ore, to bloodstone, to lodestone. These stones were used in healing in Egyptian then Chinese cultures, and later by the Greeks. In biblical times, the "laying on of hands," as practiced by Jesus, was used, transforming electromagnetic impulses from one person to another. The modern version of this technique with and without religious overtones is called therapeutic touch, healing touch, Reiki, or polarity.

In 1773, Franz Anton Mesmer used magnets for healing. His patients frequently noticed unusual currents coursing through their bodies before a healing crisis occurred. His methods were dismissed as philosophically unacceptable and by at least two scientific investigations at the time, including those by Benjamin Franklin and Antoine Laurent de Lavoisier. Magnetic healers, however, have always persisted in all cultures, including the American West, when in the 1870 s Andrew Taylor Still, the founder of osteopathy, carried a business card identifying himself as a "magnetic healer" and "lightning bone setter." The big controversy over energy healers that started with Mesmer continues today.

Mechanists vs. Vitalists

Those involved in science, medicine, and healing are basically divided into two main philosophical camps, the mechanists and vitalists. The mechanists hold that life obeys the laws of chemistry and physics, and will ultimately be totally explained by science, through the known laws of physics and chemistry. In contrast, vitalists have historically held to a belief that life will never be explained by normal laws of physics and chemistry, and that there is some kind of mysterious "life force," which is separate from the known laws of nature that distinguish living from nonliving matter.[1]

Early 19th- and 20th-century "medical" electrical therapies include the four types of electricity: static (Franklinic) energy, direct (Galvanic) current, induction-coil (Faradic) current, and high-frequency (d'Arsonval) current. Using the induction-coil method, Hugo Wilhelm von Ziemssen charted the locations of muscle points, or motor points in 1864. In 1867 Guillaume-Benjamin Duchenne published classic studies on muscle points that gave rise to the modern field of medical electromyography, in which electrical recordings are made of the activity of the muscle motor points. The Faradic current was used as therapy early in the 20th century. Today it is used diagnostically, called electromyography (EMG). EMGs are used to determine whether the muscle is properly neurologically innervated for diagnostic aids in cases of herniated discs and spinal cord injuries.

By the early 1900s, Sears Roebuck, the Chicago mass merchandiser, was selling electric belts, bands, chains, plasters, and garters that were purported to provide a quick cure for all nervous and organic disorders arising from any cause. This cure-all commercialism continued until the *Flexner Report* that was produced in 1910, which ultimately showed that electrotherapy was declared scientifically unsupportable and was legally excluded from licensed clinical medical practice.

Meanwhile, electrobiology, the scientific study of electrical effects in biological organisms, continued its advancement and progress, resulting in electricity gradually losing its mysterious connection. It became less attractive than the elusive force that the vitalists were searching for. However, this emotional dogmatic fervor persists between the mechanists and vitalists today. Currently, there is a strong academic bias against any suggestion that electrical and magnetic fields generated by tissues or organs might have any important biological purpose. They are widely thought to be mere by-products of cellular activities. However, electromagnetic medicine is beginning to revive, because of far more sophisticated science to support its contention that these electromagnetic fields have an important biological purpose in diagnosis and treatment of various disease states and the widespread development of alternative medicine practitioners, specifically hands-on therapists, describing and experiencing the "vital force."

Electromagnetic Field Investigations

Both scientists and non-scientists have been intrigued and amazed by the study of energy fields. In 1873, Edwin D. Babbitt, a minister, identified electromagnetic fields around the human body after days of living in total darkness. He drew the electron magnetic field around the head corresponding to the sights he saw in the darkness. He made a beautiful etching showing the fields of the head that he saw. His etching interestingly now corresponds to the expected neurocurrents flowing through the interhemispheric fibers of the corpus callosum of the brain.[2]

Harold Saxton Burr, PhD, Professor at Yale School of Medicine from 1929 through the 1950s, did numerous experiments and wrote papers showing the electromagnetic field in nature. During this time, Burr was researching energy fields, while most biologists and physicians were certain that any motions of energy therapy and "life/vital force" were complete nonsense. In the 1950s, Burr published a series of articles on how the electrical fields of trees change in advance of weather patterns and other atmospheric phenomena. Professor Burr was convinced that these electromagnetic fields are the basic blueprints for all living things and the electromagnetic fields reflect physical and mental characteristics. Thus, these electromagnetic forces are therefore useful for diagnostic purposes.[3]

It was physiologist Albert P. Mathews in 1903 who stated, "every excess of action, every change in the physical state of the protoplasm of any organ, or any area in the embryo or in the egg, produces, it is believed, an electrical disturbance."[4] So, not only does every event within the body, whether it is normal or pathological, produce electrical changes and charges, and alterations in electromagnetic fields within the organ and body, but also in the spaces around the body.

In the 1940s, Reinhard Voll in Germany was testing the electrical resistance of acupuncture pathways and correlating the conductance with specific pathological problems.[5] In 1973, Otto Bergsmann and Ann Woolley-Hart published a study showing that conductance of acupuncture point LR-8 was about 18 times higher in patients with known liver disease compared with those with no liver disease.[6] In 1985, S.G. Sullivan and colleagues reported that patients with lung disease had 30% lower electrical conductances at various lung points.[7] In 1996, Barbara Brewitt showed the cellular basis for viral infections, bacterial infections, and cancer affect the ionic content, water content, and pH of the extracelluar fluid, thereby affecting and influencing the cellular membrane and tissue conductances.[8]

For scientists like Burr, the link between biology and physics was not mysterious or unfathomable, or subtle. He found that biological energy is no different from any other kind of electricity, nor does it obey different laws. As a phenomenon, bioenergy fields have gone from scientific nonsense to an important and expanding subject of biomedical research. These electromagnetic fields can be detected at a distance from the body and scientists are explaining how these fields are generated and why they have become distorted when pathology is present.

Measuring Electromagnetic Fields

Since the mid-1980s, scientists have gone from a conviction that there is no such thing as energy fields in and around the human body to an absolute certainty that they exist. We now recognize that there are many forms of energy such as electric, magnetic, heat, light, electromagnetism, kinetic energy of motion, sound, gravity, vibration, elastic energy, and such. There is some fundamental principle that is present in all these forms of energy. At a fundamental level we still do not know exactly what the body electricity and magnetism really are. The electron is a basic unit and has properties such as charge, mass, and gravity, but a deeper explanation of how these properties arise is currently missing.[9] As we continue to expand scientific knowledge we continue to discover more questions regarding the fundamental unit of life; the what, where, when, how, and why.

A basic law in physics is that when an electric current flows through a conductor, a magnetic field is created in the surrounding space. This was discovered by Hans Christian Oersted in 1820. This classic law of physics was be challenged and expanded.

In 1963 Gerhard Baule and Richard McFee proved that the heart produced a strong electrical and magnetic activity, which resulted in a useful diagnostic procedure, the electrocardiogram.[10] They predicted that the heart produces magnetic fields and went on to discover with quantum physics that devices were able to pick up the field of the heart 4.5 m away from the body.

Also, in 1963, Philip Warren Anderson and John Rowell, as well as Sidney Shapiro separately, showed that something seemingly impossible could actually happen: the movement of pairs of electrons through a material (insulator).[11] This phenomenon was identified and called tunneling, something that was forbidden in the classical world of physics but easy in the quantum world. The quantum world states that classical particles, such as electrons, are at the same time waves, and waves can do things that solid particles cannot do.

Several kinds of tunneling can take place, and they are called Josephson effects. A superconducting quantum interference device or SQUID is now being used in medical research laboratories to map the biomagnetic fields produced by physiological processes inside the human body. A global network of SQUIDs is also being used to monitor movement-to-movement fluctuations in the geomagnetic field of the earth.

In 1972, David Cohen was able to extend his SQUID measurements to the fields produced by the brain.[12] These biomagnetic fields of brain measurement, "brain waves," are referred to as though they are confined to the brain but they are actually not. The electromagnetic fields of all the organs spread throughout the body and into the space around it. Thus, all forms of therapeutic contact may involve far more than simple measurement of touch-pressure on the skin and can be involved in electromagnetic forces.

What we have learned thus far is that living organisms have biomagnetic fields in and around them. These fields change from moment to moment in relation to events taking place inside the body as well as atmospheric effects upon the body. These fields give a clear presentation of what is going on in the body, from classical electrical diagnostic tools such as the electrocardiogram and the electroencephalogram to more sophisticated machines such as SQUIDs.

Electricity vs. Electronics

Biological electricity is a large-scale phenomenon arising from the movements of a charged ion such as sodium, potassium, chloride, calcium, and magnesium. In virtually all cases, the electricity arises because of the large electrical polarity across cell membranes, and the ability of these membranes to temporarily depolarize and then repolarize. Biological electronics is a relatively new subject of research. It deals with the flows of much smaller entities than ions, which result in a metabolic change/effect upon the body. These are mainly electrons, protons, and the spaces where an electron is missing, called "holes." The cytoskeleton as described next is the latticework upon which the electricity and the electronics take their effect.

Living Matrix

A few decades ago, the living cell was visualized as a membrane-bound bag containing a solution of molecules that randomly walked from one part to another and exchanged their biochemistry. Today this image is massively changing. We now know that there is very little empty space within that bag and that the cell is filled with filaments, tubes, fibers, and trabeculae, collectively called the cytoplasmic matrix or cytoskeleton. This cytoskeleton results in very little space left for a solution to be randomly diffusing and floating around. This cytoskeleton has a relationship with other cells and the extracellular matrix. This relationship is called the "trans-membrane," linking molecules or "integrins." It is recognized now that the cytoplasmic matrix also links to the nuclear envelope, nuclear matrix, and to genes. So the boundaries between the cell environment, the cell interior, and the genetic material are neither as sharp, nor as impermeable as we once thought. To put this in practical terms: what a practitioner touches is not merely the skin. One contacts the continuous interconnected webwork that extends throughout the body. Indeed, the skin is one of the first tissues in which this continuity was documented by Janice Ellison and D.R. Garrod in 1984.[13]

The discovery of neurohormones led to an understanding of how neuro- and hormonal systems interact. Chemical regulations are usually viewed in the same manner as cell metabolism, controlling substance hormones diffused through the extracellular matrix until they happen to bump into the target cells upon which they exert an influence. This imperfect view is not accepted anymore, for we know that many hormones deliver messages to the cell surfaces. This causes the production of second messages within the cells to activate the cellular activities.[14] Therefore, communications in the living system involve two languages—chemical and energetic.

These two methods of cellular communication —chemical and energetic—provide specificity and a type of reducency to the human body. The chemical regulations are carried out by hormones and various factors (growth factor, epithelial growth factor, and so on) through various second messages within the cell. There are also two kinds of energetic interactions—electrical and electronic. The electrical activities of the nerves and muscles are well known, but the electronic map of interactivity still remains to be completely discovered. "The entire living matrix is simultaneously a mechanical, vibrational or oscillatory, energetic, electronic, and informational network".[15]

The dynamics of the living matrix involve signaling and cell crawling. The molecules that link the cell interior with the extracellular matrix are called integrins, which are a class of adhesion molecules that glue cells in place. They also regulate most functions of the body. The hidden roles of integrins in arthritis, heart disease, stroke, osteoporosis, and the spread of cancer were identified by Alan Horwitz in 1997.[16] The living matrix is a dynamic rather than a fixed system with connections between adjacent cells and between the cells and the substrate.[17] "Molecules do not have to touch each other to interact. Energy can flow through the electromagnetic field. The electromagnetic field along with water forms the matrix of life." [18]

With the biochemistry taking place in a solution and the discovery of the cytoskeleton, science has advanced our understanding of solid state biochemistry. Solid state biochemistry recognizes that chemical reactions precede in a much more orderly and rapid manner if they are organized on a structural framework instead of the random walk theory. Moreover, the living matrix concept opens up the possibilities for global control: signals traveling in the matrix that can regulate or fine-tune matrix-associated enzymes throughout the organism. Messages can travel through the matrix, as by diffusion, or travel in the matrix by electronic conduction along the protein backbone. The therapeutic significance of solid state biochemistry and matrix regulation is further explained by the high degree of order, regularity, and crystallinity present in cells and tissues.[19,20]

The crystalline arrays in cells and tissues are found in a piezoelectrical fashion.[21] Piezoelectricity is a form in contradistinction to random shape; it contains parts or elements in a definite, characteristically recurrent array in space. Thus, form is the result of the orderly manner in which those elements are combined and arranged. The form of a higher order of complexity accordingly can emerge from the ordered assembly of simpler formed elements of mutual fit as stated by Paul Weiss in 1961.[22] Crystalline arrangements are the rule and not the exception in living systems.[23]

James Oschman, in 1981, stated that virtually all of the tissues in the body generate electric fields when they are compressed or stretched.[24] The piezoelectric effect is partly responsible for these electric fields. Another source of such fields is a phenomenon known as streaming potentials. When the skin is stretched or bent, as at a joint, minute electric pulsations are set up. These oscillations, and their harmonics, are precisely representative of the forces acting on the tissues involved. This information is electrically and electronically conducted through the surrounding living matrix.

Albert Szent-Györgi received the Nobel Prize in 1937 for his discovery of vitamin C, and after researching the insoluble scaffoldings of the matrix since 1941 he suggested that proteins in the body are semiconductors. He stated: "If a great number of atoms can be arranged with regularity in close proximity, as for example in a crystal lattice, single electrons cease to belong to one or two atoms only, and belong instead to the whole system. A great number of molecules may join to form energy continua, along which energy, namely excited electrons, may travel a certain distance."[25] Today we know that this is true thanks to Oschman and others.

Properties of the Living Matrix

The living matrix continuum includes all of the connective tissues (cytoskeletons) of all the cells throughout the body:

1. All of the great systems of the body are everywhere covered with material that is but a part of a continuous connective tissue fabric.
2. The connective tissues form a mechanical continuum, extending throughout the body, even into the innermost part of each cell.
3. The connective tissues determine the overall shape of the organism as well as the detailed architecture of its parts.
4. All movement of the body as a whole or of its smallest parts is created by tensions carried throughout the connective tissue fabric.
5. Each tension, each compression, each movement, causes the crystalline lattice of the connective tissues to generate bioelectronic signals that are precisely characteristic of those tensions, compressions, and movements.
6. The connective tissue fabric is a semiconducting communication network that can carry the bioelectronic signals between every part of the body and every other part.[26]

Robert O. Becker and Gary Seldon described the properties of the connective tissue layer surrounding the nervous system as the perineurium.[27] The perineurium is a distinct communication system and functions as a low voltage current, the current of injury that controls injury repair. Brain waves direct the overall operation of the nervous system and may well regulate consciousness. Becker and Seldon discovered that the perineural system is sensitive to magnetic fields. He concluded that acupuncture points and channels are input channels for the system that regulates tissue repair. In 1994, Oschman suggested that the points may be analogous to microprocessors located at nodes in a computer network[28].

Herbert Frölich discovered that living matter has a profound effect upon vibration and the vibrations directly affect the crystalline matrix. In the 1960s on the basis of quantum physics, Frölich predicted that the living matrix must produce coherent or laser-like oscillations.[29] These vibrations within the organisms occur at many different frequencies including visible and near-visible light frequencies. They are large or even gigantic in scale. Moreover, their effects are not trivial, because living matter is highly organized and exceedingly sensitive to the information conveyed by coherent signals. Coherent vibrations recognize no boundaries; they are collective or cooperative properties of the entire being. Each molecule, cell, tissue, and organ has an ideal resonant frequency that coordinates its activities.[30]

The Human Body and Energy Medicine

Donald Ingber showed how tissue, cellular, and nuclear architecture can be described as tensegrity systems.[31] He showed that the cytoskeleton behaves like a tensegrity structure. Tensegrity is a key structural, architectural, and energetic concept developed by Richard Buckminster Fuller in 1976.[32] Tensegrity concepts underlie geodesic domes, tents, and sailing vessels. It is characterized by a continuous tensional network (tendons) supported by a discontinuous set of compressive elements (struts). The basic unit is shaped as a type of isosceles triangle. This structure is seen through the human body and is constantly used in manual medicine procedures and transmitting the electromagnetic forces through out the body.[33]

In summary, in 1991, Kenneth Pienta and Donald Coffey wrote a paper entitled "Cellular harmonic information transfer through a tissue tensegrity-matrix system." It states:

> *"Cells and intracellular elements are capable of vibrating in a dynamic manner with complex harmonics, the frequency of which can now be measured and analyzed in a quantitative manner by Fourier analysis (and by other methods). Cellular events such as changes in shape, membrane ruffling, motility, and signal transduction occur within spatial and temporal harmonics that have potential regulatory importance. These vibrations can be altered by growth factors and the process of carcinogenesis. It is important to understand the mechanism by which this vibrational information is transferred directly to the cell. From these observations we propose that vibrational information is transferred through a tissue tensegrity-matrix which acts as a coupled harmonic oscillator operating as a*

signal transducing system from the cell periphery to the nucleus and ultimately to the DNA. The vibrational interactions occur through a tissue matrix system consisting of the nuclear matrix, the cytoskeleton, and the extracellular matrix that is poised to couple the biological oscillations of the cell from the peripheral membrane to the DNA through a tensegrity-matrix structure. Tensegrity has been defined as a structural system composed of discontinuous compression elements connected by continuous tension cables, which interact in a dynamic fashion. A tensegrity tissue matrix system allows for specific transfer of information through the cell, and through the organism, by direct transmission of vibrational chemomechanical energy through harmonic wave motion."[34]

Oschman hypothesized:

"Every part of the body, including all of the molecules so thoroughly studied by modern science, as well as the acupuncture meridians of traditional East Asian or Oriental medicine, forms a continuously interconnected semiconductor electronic network. Each component of the organism, even the smallest part, is immersed in, and generates, a constant stream of vibratory information. This is information about all of the activities taking place everywhere in the body.

Complete health corresponds to total interconnectedness. Accumulated physical and/or emotional traumas impair the connections. When this happens, the body's defense and repair systems become impaired and disease has a chance to take hold. Acupuncture and other energy therapies restore and balance the vibratory circuitry, with obvious and profound benefits. This enables the body's defense and repair systems to repair themselves.

Many individuals, both scientists and therapists, have contributed valuable insights to this emerging picture of how the body functions in health and disease. Phenomena that previously seemed disconnected and unrelated are now complementing one another, giving us a more complete understanding than we could have obtained through any single approach."[35]

YNSA and Energy Medicine

How does what we now know about electromagnetic fields, vibrational chemomechanical energy, and harmonic wavemotion provide any benefit in utilizing YNSA? What the author suggests is a simple way to prove that prior to placement of the needle in the scalp the practitioner has found the correct quadrant and the exact point that will be effective. One way to see this work is to palpate and elicit a YNSA diagnosis tender point. Then place one finger from the other hand over the proper YNSA acupoint. The result will be YNSA neck diagnosis tenderness pain relief immediately. This is the bioenergetic procedure. What is interesting now is that we are able to use these electromagnetic fields in healing as described by others in the field of Reiki and others, and those of us using YNSA have provided both a palpatory bioenergetic diagnostic method and a therapeutic bioenergetic treatment, all providing an immediate feedback mechanism. The key use of this bioenergetic healing method is in refining your diagnosis and improving your specificity of YNSA needle placement and needle manipulation in treatment.

The common dilemma the practitioner has in using the YNSA diagnostic method is: Is the sternocleidomastoid (SCM) in Procedure 2 (see p. 58) hard or soft? Or more specifically, do I interpret the tissue feel of the SCM Yin of YIN, Yang of YANG, Yin of YANG, or Yang of YIN? The solution is to employ the bioenergetic procedure for proper quadrant identification.

Bioenergetic Procedure

The YNSA bioenergetic procedure is often used for proper quadrant identification, is: With one hand identify the Ypsilon tender point. HT, GB, or LR are typically the best because they are commonly found and easily identified in ALL four quadrants. With the other hand place the index finger on the Ypsilon point starting in the Yin of YIN quadrant. If the neck Ypsilon tenderness goes away, one has correctly identified the right quadrant to treat. Move in this order of importance starting with Yin of YIN, then Yang of YIN, then Yin of YANG, and finally, Yang of YANG until pain relief is achieved.

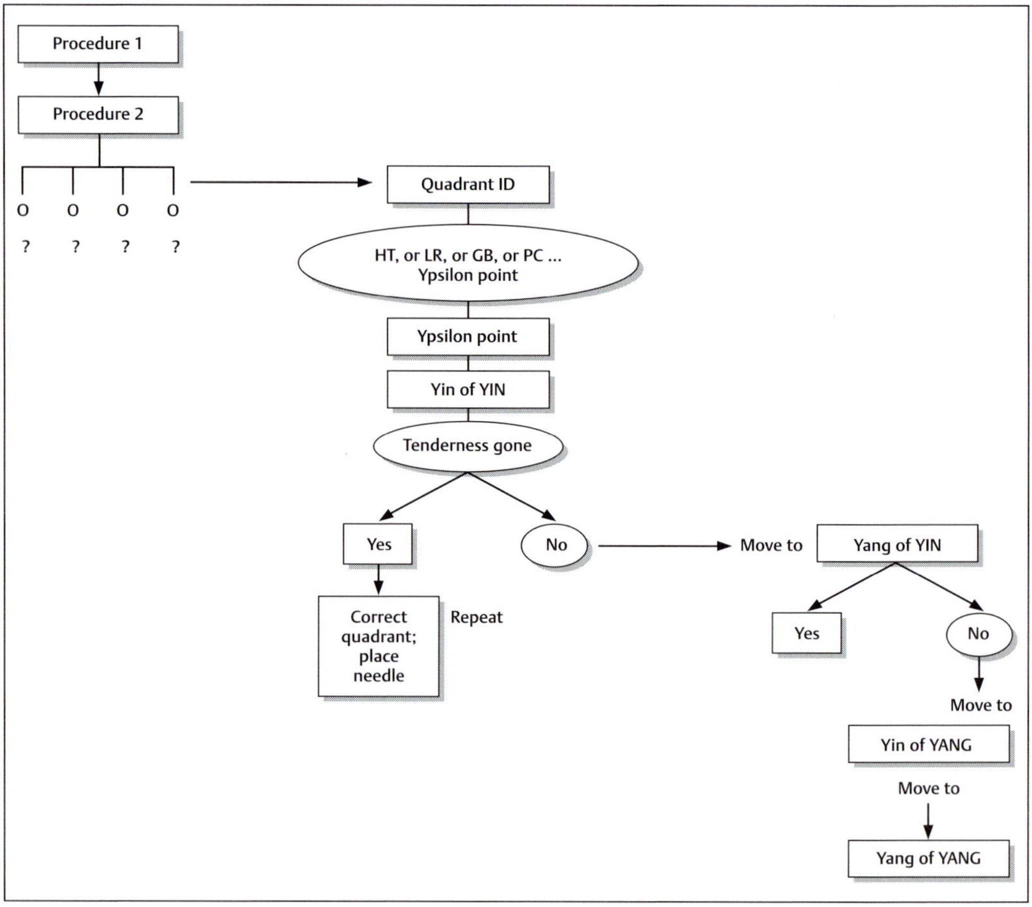

Figure 3–1 Energetic procedure of quadrant identification.

To summarize:
Energetic procedure of quadrant identification (**Figure 3–1**):

1. Palpate the tender YNSA neck diagnosis Ypsilon point and maintain pressure.
2. Practitioners' opposite hand, index finger only, is placed on the corresponding scalp Ypsilon point starting with Yin of YIN, moving to Yang of YIN, then Yin of YANG, and finally to Yang of YANG until there is no tenderness in the neck diagnosis Ypsilon point.

Final Thoughts

It has been scientifically proven that there are pathways involved in electromagnetic reception within the body and the cells. We have identified that there is regulation of the brain waves and therapeutic emissions from the hands of manual therapists. We have identified micropulsations of the geomagnetic fields caused by Schumann resonance, which are detected by the pineal gland and magnetite-bearing tissues associated with the brain.[36,37] The human resonance can take over as a pacemaker and particularly if the individual is in a relaxed or a meditative state. These human signals are thousands of times stronger than brain waves. The brain waves regulate the overall tone of the nervous system and the state of consciousness. The electrical currents of brain waves are conducted throughout the body by the perineural and vascular systems. The biomagnetic field projected from the hands can be much stronger than the brain waves, according to Asaka Seto and colleagues, 1992, which indicated that an amplification of at least 1000 times takes place somewhere in the body.[38] Alternatively, the body may simply act as an effective antenna or channel for the human micropulsations. The projected fields scan or sweep through the frequencies, which medical researchers are finding useful for jumpstarting injury repair in a variety of tissues. Thus, we have identified that the earth has an electromagnetic field, which causes human resonance, influences the pineal gland and magnetic-bearing tissues, effectively modulating in the brain alpha waves.[39] This then stimulates the perineural system and is transmitted through the hands by a projected biomagnetic field to result in injury repair of the tissues. We can now show that an individual cell fits into the acupuncture channel scheme with the cytoskeleton as the main structure affecting the cell and the nervous system, fitting together in a complex matrix.[40] This matrix relies upon the tensegrity structure for architectural shape and energetic function allowing coherent harmonic vibrations to resonate. The channel system used in acupuncture describes the channel branching into every part of the organism through the perineural network electrically extending into the interior of every cell through the cytoskeleton and crystalline structures of the body and even into the nuclei containing genetic materials. These acupuncture channels are simply the main channels or transmission lines in the continuous molecular fabric of the body.[41] The molecular web is both a mechanical/anatomical structure as well as vibratory network with electrical and electronic transmission that has a profound biological and clinical significance.[42]

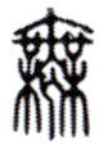 ䷊ 泰 ***Taí***

Advance—Earth and Heaven Unite

"Advance.
The little is departing;
The great is arriving.
Good fortune.
Prosperous and smooth.
Heaven and Earth unite;
All beings come into union.
The upper and the lower link;
Their wills are the same.
The inner is the yang; *the outer is the* yin.
The inner is the strong; the outer is the gentle.
The inner is the superior; the outer is the inferior.
Thus,
The way of the superior is expanding;
The way of the inferior is shrinking."[43]

References

1. Becker RO, Matino AA. Electromagnetism and Life. Albany: State University of New York Press; 1982
2. Oschman JL. Energy Medicine: The Scientific Basis. Edinburgh: Churchill Livingstone; 2000: 12
3. Oschman JL. Energy Medicine: The Scientific Basis. Edinburgh: Churchill Livingstone; 2000: 16–18
4. Mathews AP. Electric polarity in hydroids. American Journal of physiology 1903;8: 294–299
5. Voll R. The phenomenon of medicine testing in electro-acupuncture according to Voll. American Journal of Acupuncture 1980;8: 97–104.
6. Bergsmann O, Woolley-Hart A. Differences in electrical skin conductivity between acupuncture points and adjacent skin areas. American Journal of Acupuncture 1973;1: 27–32
7. Sullivan SG, Eggleston W, Martinoff JT, Kroenig RJ. Evoked electrical conductivity on the lung acupuncture points in healthy individuals and confirmed lung cancer patients. American Journal of Acupuncture 1985;13(3):261–266
8. Brewitt B. Quantitative analysis of electrical skin conductance in diagnosis: historical and current views of bioelectrical medicine. Journal of Naturopathic Medicine 1996;6(1):66–75
9. Oschman JL. Energy Medicine in Therapeutics and Human Performance. St. Louis: Butterworth-Heinemann; 2003: 47

10. Baule GM, McFee R. Detection of the magnetic field of the heart. American Heart Journal 1963;66: 95–96
11. Anderson PW, Rowell JM. Probable observation of the Josephson superconducting tunneling effect. *Physical Review Letters* 1963;10: 230–232
12. Cohen D. Magnetoencephalography: detection of the brain's electrical activity with a superconducting magnetometer. Science 1972;175: 664–666
13. Ellison J, Garrod DR. Anchoring filaments of the amphibian epidural junction transverse the basal lamina entirely from the plasma membrane of hemidesmosomes to the dermis. *Journal of Cell Science* 1984;72: 163–172
14. Rasmussen H. Calcium and cAMP as Synarchic Messengers. New York: John Wiley and Sons; 1981
15. Pienta KJ, Coffey DS. Cellular harmonic information transfer through a tissue tensegrity-matrix system. Medical Hypotheses 1991;34: 88–95
16. Horwitz AF. Integrins and health. Discovered only recently, these adhesive cell surface molecules have quickly revealed themselves to be critical to proper functioning of the body and to life itself. Scientific American 1997;276: 68–75
17. Szent-Györgi A. Bioelectronics. New York: Academic Press; 1968
18. Szent-Györgi A. Bioelectronics. New York: Academic Press; 1957: 139
19. Ho M-W. Coherent energy, liquid crystallinity and acupuncture, talk presented to British Acupuncture Society, October 2, 1999. Available at: http://www.i-sis.org.uk/acupunc.php. Accessed September 4, 2009
20. Ho M-W. The acupuncture system and the liquid crystalline collegen fibers of the connective tisues. American Journal of Chinese Medicine 1998;26: 251–263
21. Bassett CAL, Becker RO. Generation of electrical potentials by bone in response to mechanical stress. Science 1962;137: 1063–1064
22. Weiss PA. Biological foundation of wound repair. Harvey Lectures 1961;55: 13–42
23. Weiss PA. The science of life: the living system–a system for living. In: Shaefer KE, Hensel H, Brady R (editors). A New Image of Man in Medicine, Volume I, Toward a Man-centered Medical Science. Mount Kisco, NY: Futura Publishing Company; 1977
24. Oschman JL. The connective tissue and myofascial systems. In: Readings on the Scientific Basis of Bodywork, Energetic, and Movement Therapies. Dover, NH: NORA Press; 1981
25. Szent-Györgi A. Bioelectronics. New York: Academic Press; 1968
26. Oschman JL. Energy Medicine in Therapeutics and Human Performance. St. Louis: Butterworth-Heinemann; 2003: 55
27. Becker RO, Seldon G. The Body Electric: Electromagnetism and the Foundation of Life. New York: William Morrow and Company; 1985
28. Oschman JL, Oschman NH. New evidence on the nature of healing energy. Part 1: Communication in the living matrix. Dover: NORA Press; 1994
29. Frohlich H. Quantum mechanical concepts in biology. In: Marios M (editor). Theoretical Physics and Biology. Amsterdam: North Holland; 1969
30. Frohlich H, Kremer F. Coherent Excitations in Biological Systems. New York: Springer-Verlag; 1983
31. Ingber DE. The riddle of morphogenesis: a question of solution chemistry or molecular cell engineering? Cell 1993;75: 1249–1252
32. Pugh A. An Introduction to Tensegrity. Berkeley: University of California Press; 1976
33. Oschman JL. Energy Medicine in Therapeutics and Human Performance. St. Louis: Butterworth-Heinemann; 2003: 63
34. Pienta KJ, Coffey DS. Cellular harmonic information transfer through a tissue tensetrity-matrix system. Medical Hypotheses 1991;34: 88–95
35. Oschman JL. Energy Medicine: The Scientific Basis. Edinburgh: Churchill Livingstone; 2000: 71
36. Schlegel K, Fuellekrug M. 50 Years of Schumann Resonance (translated by Catarina Geoghan in 2007). Originally published in *Physik in unserer Zeit* 2002;33(6):256–261
37. Oschman JL. Energy Medicine: The Scientific Basis. Edinburgh: Churchill Livingstone; 2000: 99
38. Seto A, Kusaka C, Nakazato S, Huang W, Sato T, Hisamitsu T, Takeshige C. Detection of extraordinary large biomagnetic field strength from human hand during external *qi* emission. Acupuncture and Electro-therapeutics Research International Journal 1992;17: 75–94
39. Oschman JL. Energy Medicine: The Scientific Basis. Edinburgh: Harcourt Brace/Churchill Livingstone; 2000
40. Ingber DE. The riddle of morphogenesis: a question of solution chemistry or molecular cell engineering? Cell 1993;75: 1249–1252
41. Myers T. Anatomy Trains. Myofascial Meridians for Manual and Movement Therapists. Edinburgh: Churchill Livingstone; 2001
42. Oschman JL. Energy Medicine: The Scientific Basis. Edinburgh: Churchill Livingstone; 2000: 70
43. Huang A. The Complete I Ching Rochester, VT: Inner Traditions; 1998: 118–119

4

YNSA Indications, Contraindications, and Side Effects

"The sages do not treat those who have already fallen ill, but rather those who are not yet ill."

"When medical therapy is initiated only after someone has fallen ill, … it is as though someone has waited to dig a well until he is already weak with thirst. Is this not too late?"—Huang-di Nei-jing Su-wen

"YNSA is a fast acting, reliable, time-saving method for treatment of many types of illnesses, disabilities, and painful conditions."[1] – Toshikatsu Yamamoto, MD, PhD

Indications for YNSA

The indications for the use of YNSA in patients are many. The requirements for the use of YNSA include:

- Positive history for disease, trauma, dysfunction, pain, or illness that could be benefited by the use of acupuncture or YNSA.
- Finding a positive YNSA neck, abdomen, or pulse diagnosis is necessary to determine which particular YNSA acupuncture point (acupoint) is needed regardless of whether treatment is required for disease or prevention.

Thus, armed with these two requirements, the practitioner may try to improve health, alleviate dysfunction, and/or resolve disease. In conjunction with a cooperative patient without contraindications, the trained, licensed practitioner may now begin to use YNSA.

The medical and surgical indications for YNSA are many and diverse. In clinical cases, YNSA has been used to treat hundreds of various diseases. These include organ and systemic diseases and/or dysfunction affecting the musculoskeletal, neurological, psychological, genitourinary, digestive, circulatory, respiratory, cardiovascular, endocrine, and immune systems and special senses. Good success is routinely achieved with neurological and musculoskeletal disorders with the use of YNSA as either a primary or complementary treatment. These disorders include headache, neuritis, neuropathies, migraine, trigeminal neuralgia, Meniere's disease, Bell's palsy, other entrapment neuropathies, intercostal neuralgia, adhesive capsulitis, tennis elbow, sciatica, low back pain, rheumatoid arthritis, osteoarthritis, and radiculopathies of the cervical and lumbar spine. YNSA has been quite effective as a complementary treatment of both chronic and acute pain.[2] Some other conditions where YNSA has been helpful include: upper motor neuron loss or lesions resulting in dysfunction, lower motor loss or lesions resulting in dysfunction, sensory loss and dysfunctions, neuroendocrine dysfunctions and disease, and visceral dysfunctions and disease. Obviously, only a few YNSA treatments cannot change anatomical lesions or structure pathology such as tumors or blood clots.

The indications for YNSA as primary treatment include all acute pain conditions if no anatomical underlying cause is known. It is amazing how rapidly proper YNSA needle placement in the scalp will cause acute pain to immediately abate. Other indications for YNSA treatment that may be either primary or complementary are summarized in **Table 2–14** in Chapter 2.

YNSA's most dramatic effect is in the treatment of pain, dysfunction, and neurological diseases. Finally, YNSA is indicated when a positive YNSA neck or YNSA abdominal diagnosis is found. If you do not find positive findings upon standard medical physical examination, TCM examination, or YNSA neck or abdominal diagnosis findings, then YNSA is not indicated.

Contraindications for YNSA

There are very few contraindications for a trained YNSA physician and a willing patient to participate in this form of medical acupuncture. The primary responsibility of the physician is to make a medical diagnosis with particular attention to the neuromusculoskeletal and visceral systems. Following a history, physical, and acupuncture (YNSA and/or TCM [Eight Principles and/or Five Phases]) examination, a working diagnosis is made. YNSA may then be used as a therapeutic means to alleviate pain and suffering and to improve physiological function. With that being said, the contraindications to YNSA include:

- Systemic infection and certain critically ill patients
- Needling into a scalp skin infection or ulceration
- Needling over a fontanelle or where the cranial bone has been surgically removed
- Negative TCM or YNSA diagnostic procedures

Situations where YNSA requires caution and/or restraint are the following: forceful manipulation of the needle, patients with organic or iatrogenic bleeding conditions, pregnant women, patients with previous needle shock, young children, infants, and neonates. Concern needs to be taken regarding the patient's physical, psychological, and nutritional status. The following patients should probably not be treated according to TCM tradition, which is in agreement with YNSA:

- Those on an empty stomach, fasting for more than 12 hours
- Those very emotionally agitated
- Those on street drugs or alcohol
- Those who have just engaged in extreme physical excitement[3]

High-Risk Patient Conditions[3]

- Positive cardiac disease or abnormal heart valves
- HIV+
- Receiving radiation or chemotherapy for cancer
- Severe complicated diabetes
- Pregnancy
- Systemic lupus erythematosus
- Asthma
- Hypertension
- Cerebrovascular accident (CVA), transient ischemic attack (TIA)

Precautions and Advice

Although acupuncture is safe and relatively free of side effects, some accidents take place owing to negligence by the physician, the patient's condition(s), contraindications, and/or imperfect needle manipulations. High-risk does not equal contraindication to YNSA treatment. It is important that the YNSA physician be experienced and have knowledge, skill, and ability in treatment of complications associated with any acupuncture treatment, particularly YNSA. One must be familiar with the location of major blood vessels in the scalp to avoid puncturing them, particularly with those patients on anticoagulants. One must be cognizant of patients with previous needle shock. Due care and caution must be maintained, especially when acupuncturing young children. When treating pregnant women, certain YNSA points should be avoided, particularly those relating to and involving the abdomen, low back, sacral region, spleen, large intestine, stomach, and bladder. Ypsilon points should be refrained from use after the first trimester of pregnancy. The YNSA physician should follow the *Inner Canon*, which warns against performing acupuncture within an hour before and after a patient may have had sexual intercourse, eaten a large meal, drunk alcohol, become exhausted, or traveled a long distance, or if the patient is in a state of fright or anger. There is no known indication for moxa on any of the YNSA points; electrical stimulation to the YNSA points is not used.

Complications and Common Side Effects

Complications to acupuncture include needle shock, fatigue, nausea, pain, bleeding, and seizure. The most common side effect is bleeding after the needle is removed, followed by pain. Less common is needle shock and nausea. The least common is seizure. Extremely rare possibilities are cardiovascular complications, myocardial infarction, and cardiac arrest.

Cardiovascular Complications

Cardiovascular complications are very rare. In all cases, remove needles and place patient supine. In rare cases angina may result, if licensed treat and contact EMS or 911.[4]

- *Myocardial infarction.* Very rare. Contact EMS or 911 to transport patient to the emergency room.
- *Cardiac arrest.* Very rare. Contact EMS or 911 and begin administering CPR.
- *Fainting.* Uncommon. Treat with smelling salts, or GV-26.5.
- *Vasovagal response.* Not uncommon. Treat supine, with blankets to keep warm.
- *Epistaxis.* Rare. To treat, apply pressure at the soft lobular part of the nostrils with clean gauze. Tilt head backwards.

Iatrogenic Complications

- *Forgotten needles.* Not uncommon. Keep a count of needles in place in all patients to verify when removing.
- *Broken needle.* Rare. If the shaft is above the skin, remove with a sterile hemostat; if the shaft is below the skin, surgical referral for removal by surgeon is necessary.

- *Blood vessel puncture.* Not uncommon. If a small superficial vein, mild pressure for about 1 minute. After removal of the needle, hematoma will develop. If a small artery, apply firm pressure for 3 to 5 minutes. If a large artery, apply firm pressure for 10 to 30 minutes.[5]
- *Neuralgia.* Not uncommon. Remove needle and apply ice for 15 minutes.

It is normal for patients to experience pain when the needle goes in as well as for a short time (10 to 30 seconds) after it is inserted. If the patient feels uncomfortable after that time, the best management is to withdraw the needle slightly to regulate the depth and angle of insertion. If pain still persists, the needle should be removed. To prevent needle shock from the first treatment, use YNSA with the patient supine. The younger the patient, particularly preteen and teen males, the greater the likelihood for needle shock to occur. Needle shock can be reversed by:

- Removal of all needles
- Having the patient supine
- Smelling salts
- Use of the following body acupoints: GV-26.5 and/or KI-1; LI-4 and/or ST-36

To prevent bleeding, use a cottonball when pulling out the needle from the scalp. Closing the hole afterward with digital pressure is usually quite effective. Using YNSA on patients taking blood-thinning medications requires precaution when removing the needles but YNSA may and can be used.

For persistent pain after the needle has been removed, the recommended treatment is an ice cube to the needled area for 15 minutes. Fatigue posttreatment is due to overtreatment—too many needles or needles left in scalp for longer than 20 minutes. To prevent fatigue, use fewer needles, especially for the first few visits.

Patients should be told that scalp acupuncture is commonly associated with transient pain upon placement of the needle (10 to 30 seconds). Furthermore, educate the patient as to where the needle is to be inserted into the skin, not the brain or bone, to allay fear. A calm, professional demeanor and appropriate explanations and expectations will help the patient understand the procedure and goals of treatment. Normal side effects include euphoria, mild disorientation, transient dizziness, and lightheadedness.

Summary

YNSA is quite effective for acute and chronic pain. It is indicated for all World Health Organization acupuncture indications and many other conditions. It is contraindicated in cases of severe infection, and precautions should be taken with children, adolescents, and pregnant women.

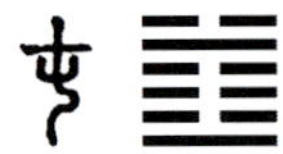 屯 ***Zhún***

Beginning—Cloud Above, Thunder Below

"Beginning. The firm and the yielding
united at the very beginning;
Difficulties come into being.
Movement in the midst
of danger, Great prosperity and
smoothness comes through steadfastness
and uprightness."[6]

"After Heaven and Earth have come
into existence, myriad beings are
produced. These myriad beings fill up
the space between Heaven and Earth.
Thus, Beginning follows."[7]

References

Additional references are available on page 148.

1. Yamamoto T, Yamamoto H. Yamamoto New Scalp Acupuncture (YNSA). Tokyo, Japan: Axel Springer Japan Publishing, Inc.; 1998: 17
2. Yamamoto T, Yamamoto H. Yamamoto New Scalp Acupuncture (YNSA). Tokyo, Japan: Axel Springer Japan Publishing, Inc.; 1998: 11
3. Belluomini J. Clean Needle Technique: A Manual for Acupuncturists. Brookline, MA: Complementary Medicine Press; 1999: 61
4. Belluomini J. Clean Needle Technique: A Manual for Acupuncturists. Brookline, MA: Complementary Medicine Press; 1999: 35–39
5. Belluomini J. Clean Needle Technique: A Manual for Acupuncturists. Brookline, MA: Complementary Medicine Press; 1999: 41–45
6. Huang A. The Complete I Ching. Rochester, VT: Inner Traditions; 1998: 58
7. Huang A. The Complete I Ching. Rochester, VT: Inner Traditions; 1998: 57

5

YNSA Neck Diagnosis Points

"What is to be reduced is first expanded.

What is to be weakened is first strengthened.

What is to be abolished is first established."[1]

"He who asks is a fool for five minutes but he who does not ask remains a fool forever." – Chinese Proverb

YNSA. YNSA is a diagnosis and treatment microsystem utilizing the YNSA neck diagnosis procedure for anatomical and channel dysfunction or disease. The anatomical system uses Basic points, and a channel system uses Ypsilon points.

YNSA neck diagnosis. The unique palpatory examination of the neck soft tissue structures as developed by Dr. Yamamoto to identify axial skeletal and channel dysfunction, vacuity, or repletion.

This chapter discusses the methods and procedures of doing YNSA neck diagnosis. It is critical to master YNSA neck diagnosis to know which Basic and Ypsilon points to treat; see **Figure 5–1** to review the steps in diagnosis and treatment. It is necessary to master which phase to treat, either YIN or YANG and either left and/or right. In all cases where YNSA is considered or used, YNSA neck and/or abdominal diagnosis procedures should be used. **Figures 5–2 and 5–3** encapsulate the procedures for determining sidedness (first procedure), phase YIN or YANG (second procedure), quadrant (third procedure), and Basic points.

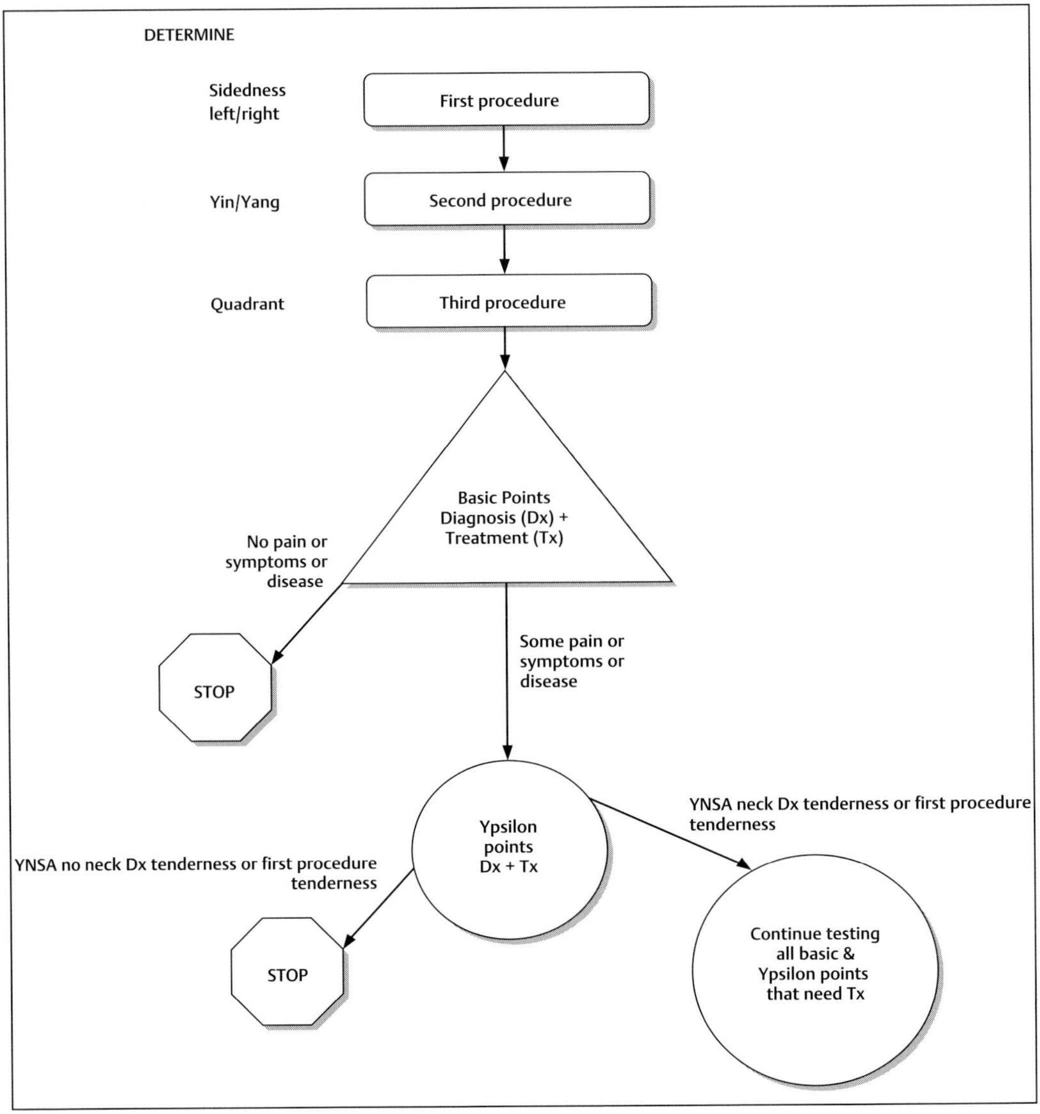

Figure 5–1 YNSA diagnosis and treatment.

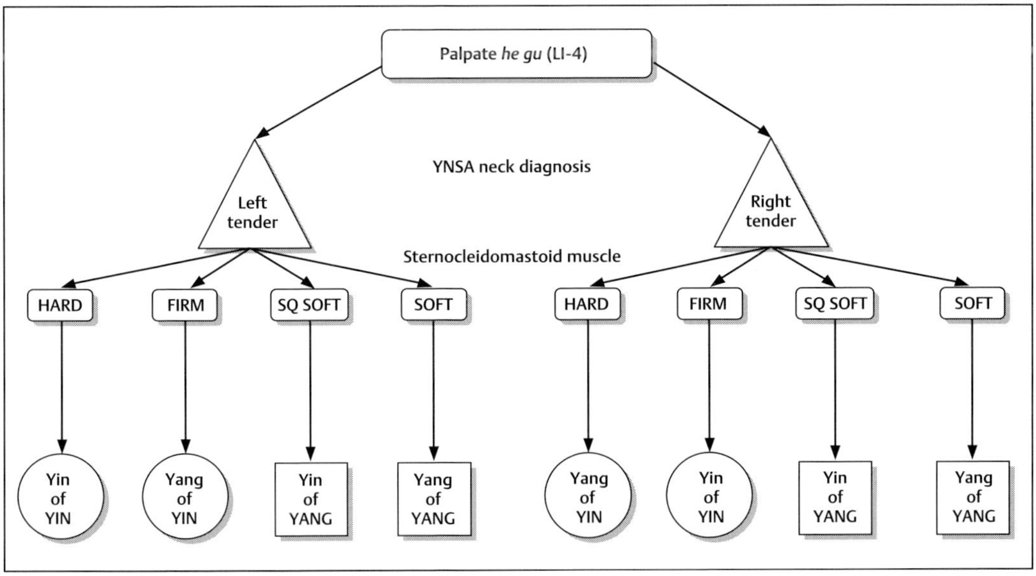

Figure 5–2 YNSA neck diagnosis.

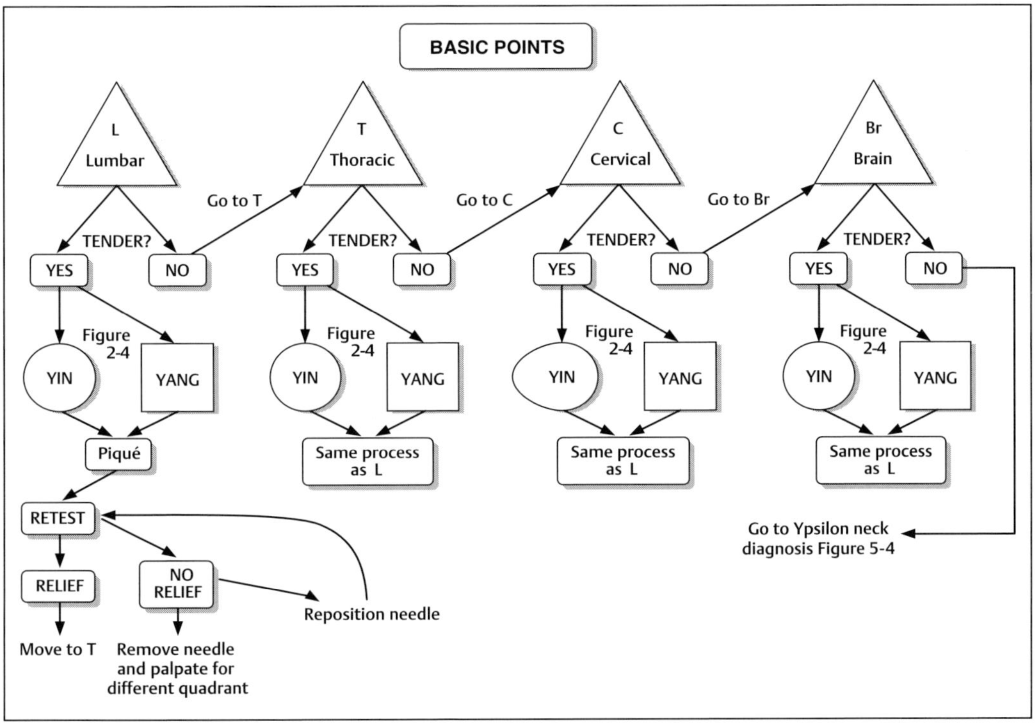

Figure 5–3 YNSA Basic point diagnosis.

YNSA Neck Diagnosis Principles

First Procedure. Sidedness: To Determine Sidedness, Left or Right

Purpose

Determine sidedness for neck diagnostic testing

Method

1. Have the patient sitting facing the physician standing.
2. Grasp the patient's left hand with your right hand.
3. Compress the patient's LI-4, *he gu*, points with your thumbs.
4. Ask the patient which is most tender.
5. The most tender side indicates the sidedness or the side that needs treatment first.

Second Procedure. Phase: To Determine YIN or YANG

Purpose

Determine whether you need to treat in YIN or YANG.

Method

1. Place thumb over liver (LR) neck diagnosis spot on the sternocleidomastoid muscle (SCM).
2. Compress LR point with thumb and rub back and forth on the SCM.
3. Result: YIN is soft to palpation, therefore treat in YANG.
4. Result: YANG is hard and firm to palpation, therefore treat in YIN.

Third Procedure. Quadrant: Ypsilon Neck Diagnosis Procedure To Verify Correct Quadrant

YNSA is based on the systematic correspondences associated with the four quadrants—Yin of YIN, Yang of YIN, Yin of YANG, and Yang of YANG—which are key in determining correct needle placement and achieving excellent results using YNSA. See **Figure 5–4** for delineation of specific points.

Purpose

To determine correct quadrant for needle placement after the first and second procedures are done.

Method

1. Determine sidedness of neck diagnosis using first procedure.
2. Determine YIN or YANG using second procedure.
3. Palpate the SCM at the level of the Liver (LR), slide the thumb back and forth pressing posterior medially for several seconds (30–40 seconds). If the liver (LR) is tender (positive) move to step 4. If the liver (LR) is not tender (negative), move to PC, HT, GB, and KI, in that order, to identify a tender (positive) Ypsilon point.
4. Identify a positive YNSA neck diagnosis Ypsilon point on the correct side in the correct quadrant.
   Bioenergetic procedure: With one thumb on the positive YNSA neck diagnosis Ypsilon tender point, place the other hand's index finger over the scalp Ypsilon point, if the second procedure identified YIN, first try Yin of YIN to see if tenderness diminishes. If tenderness goes away, one has successfully found the correct quadrant to treat. If it is still tender, move index finger to Yang of YIN. The tenderness should go away when the finger is on the exact point in the correct quadrant. The same procedure may be applied in the YANG quadrants if the second procedure identified YANG.
5. Next, piqué the Ypsilon point on the correct side in the correct quadrant. Retest neck tender point; if normal (nontender), then one has found the right quadrant (phase) end point, continue with the rest of the treatment. If the tender point does not improve, recheck the needling technique. Remove the needle and replace it in the correct Ypsilon point in the corresponding quadrant.
6. Once the correct quadrant is identified, by tradition all positive Basic points are piquéd first and then any remaining Ypsilon points are taken.

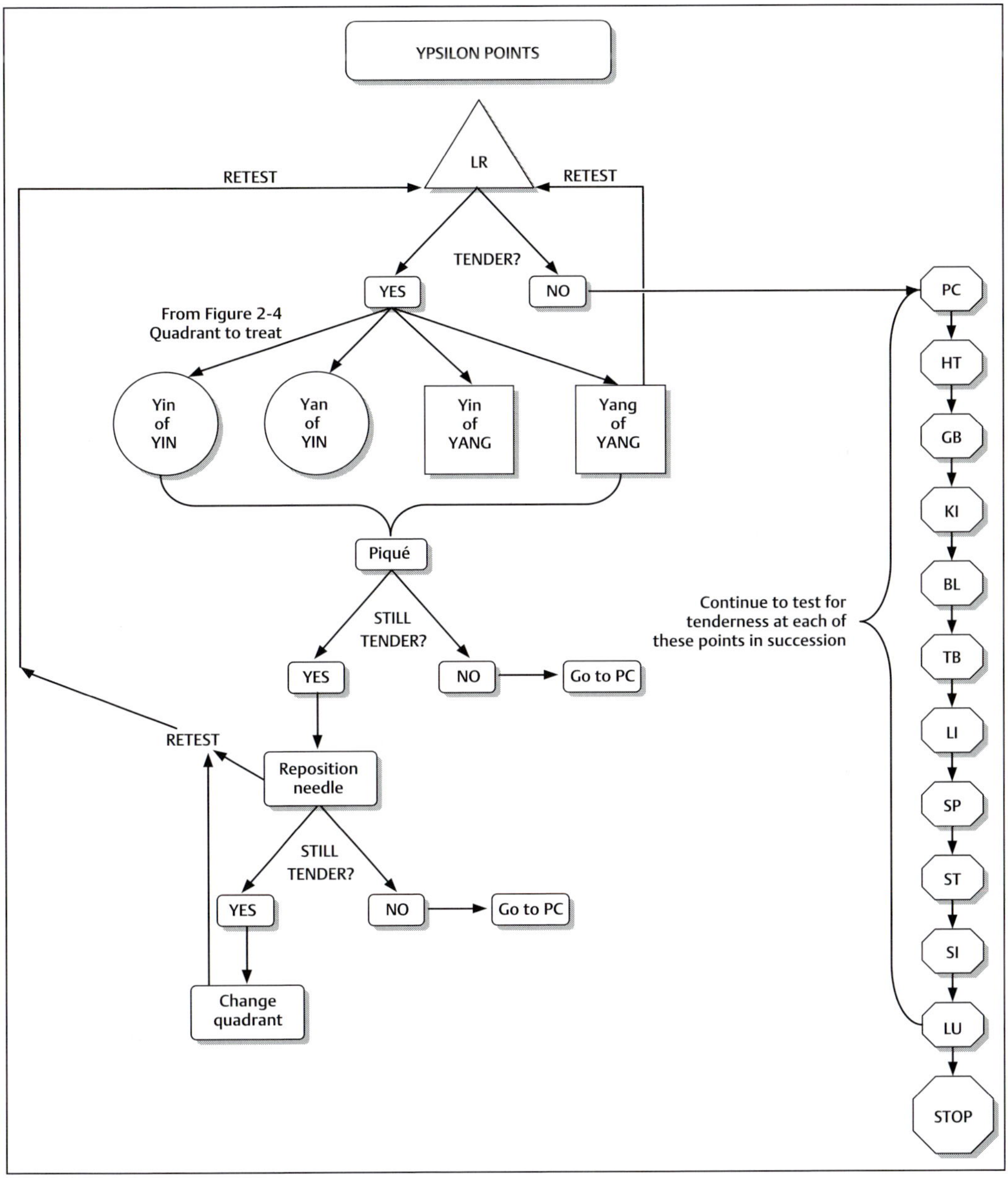

Figure 5–4 YNSA Ypsilon point diagnosis.

YNSA Basic Neck Diagnosis Systematic Procedure

Procedure

YNSA basic point neck diagnosis: to diagnose by palpation the anatomical structures related to the spine and the central nervous system. Basic points may be used for a myriad of conditions that relate medically and physiologically to these structures. The YNSA basic neck diagnosis tests for lumbar spine, thoracic spine, cervical spine, and brain Basic points.

Purpose

To determine if the spine and brain points are positive (tender) needing treatment.

Method

1. Place thumb on the most tender side as detected by the First Procedure, LI-4 testing, over the lumbar neck diagnosis point—located over the first rib between the anterior scalene and the SCM. Press medial to determine tenderness. LI-14 is an alarm point for upper body problems, but I find it is also tender for the lower body.
2. Then test the thoracic spine, one thumb breadth lateral to lumbar, then cervical, again one thumb breadth lateral, and finally the brain points, which are one thumb breadth lateral to the cervical point.
3. Rank these points in order of tenderness, with the most severe first.
4. Treat the most tender point first, then retest that point to determine if it has improved.
5. Retest other positive (tender) basic neck points and treat.
6. Then test basic diagnosis points on the other side of the neck.
7. Treat only the positive tender points first, then one may secondarily treat anatomically related points based on history.
8. After one has diagnosed and treated all of the positive Basic points related to the patient's condition, if symptoms still persist move on to Ypsilon neck diagnosis. If the patient does not have any symptoms, stop.

YNSA Ypsilon Neck Diagnosis Systematic Procedure

Procedure

The Ypsilon neck diagnosis systematic procedure is a quick and systematic way of performing YNSA neck diagnosis. It was developed and refined to be used with the least amount of motion and the most reliability and reproducibility in palpating for tenderness over the correct anatomical locations. **Figure 5–5** delineates all the YNSA neck diagnosis tender points and **Figure 5–6** identifies the anatomical structures that one needs to be cognizant of during the YNSA neck diagnosis palpation, particularly the SCM, both heads of the SCM as it attaches to the manibrium sterni and the clavicle, the trapezius muscle, the posterior scalene and scalenus muscles, and the omohyoid muscle.

Method

1. After one has done the first procedure, the correct side to diagnose and treat has been identified. The physician is facing the seated patient and places his thumb over the patient's SCM. For example, when the patient sidedness is left, the physician's right thumb is used.
2. Placing the thumb over the belly of the SCM, at the level of the thyroid cartilage, press the thumb posterior medially maintaining contact over the SCM, sliding back and forth to elicit tenderness. If tenderness is elicited upon questioning, it is considered a positive liver (LR) Ypsilon point and will require YNSA Ypsilon treatment. If it is not tender, move to the next Ypsilon point.
3. From the liver (LR), curl the thumb anterior medial and posterior over the edge of the SCM and press posteriorly to elicit tenderness. If there is tenderness, then one has a positive pericardium (PC) YNSA neck diagnosis tender point.
4. From the pericardium (PC), slide the thumb superior one thumb breadth up the anterior belly of the SCM to palpate the heart (HT). Press posterior to elicit tenderness.
5. From the heart (HT), slide the thumb caudad along the anterior belly of the SCM past the pericardium (PC) to one finger breadth below the pericardium (PC) tender point. This is gall bladder (GB). Press posterior to elicit tenderness.
6. It is at this point that YNSA needle treatment usually begins. First piqué the scalp YNSA points in the correct quadrant from the most to the least tender, in that order, based on the neck diagnosis procedures above.
7. From the gall bladder (GB), move the thumb off the SCM and place it between the mandibular and clavicular heads of SCM just superior to the clavicle. In that triangular hole, press the thumb posteriorly. This is kidney (KI). If tender it is positive and needs to be treated on the scalp.
8. From kidney (KI), rotate the thumb so that the thumbnail is pointed caudally and inferior and just posterior to the clavicle. Pressing caudally, this is the bladder (BL). If tender, it is positive and needs to be treated.
9. From bladder (BL), move the thumb to the trapezius, 4 finger breadths (3 cun) lateral to the

root of the neck over the trapezius muscle to search the next group of points. The first point is underneath the roll of the trapezius muscle and posteriorly one will find the triple burner (TB). If tender, it is positive and needs to be treated.

10. From the triple burner (TB), on top of the trapezius muscle at that same location and pressing caudally on top of the trapezius roll, is the large intestine (LI). If tender, it is positive and needs to be treated.

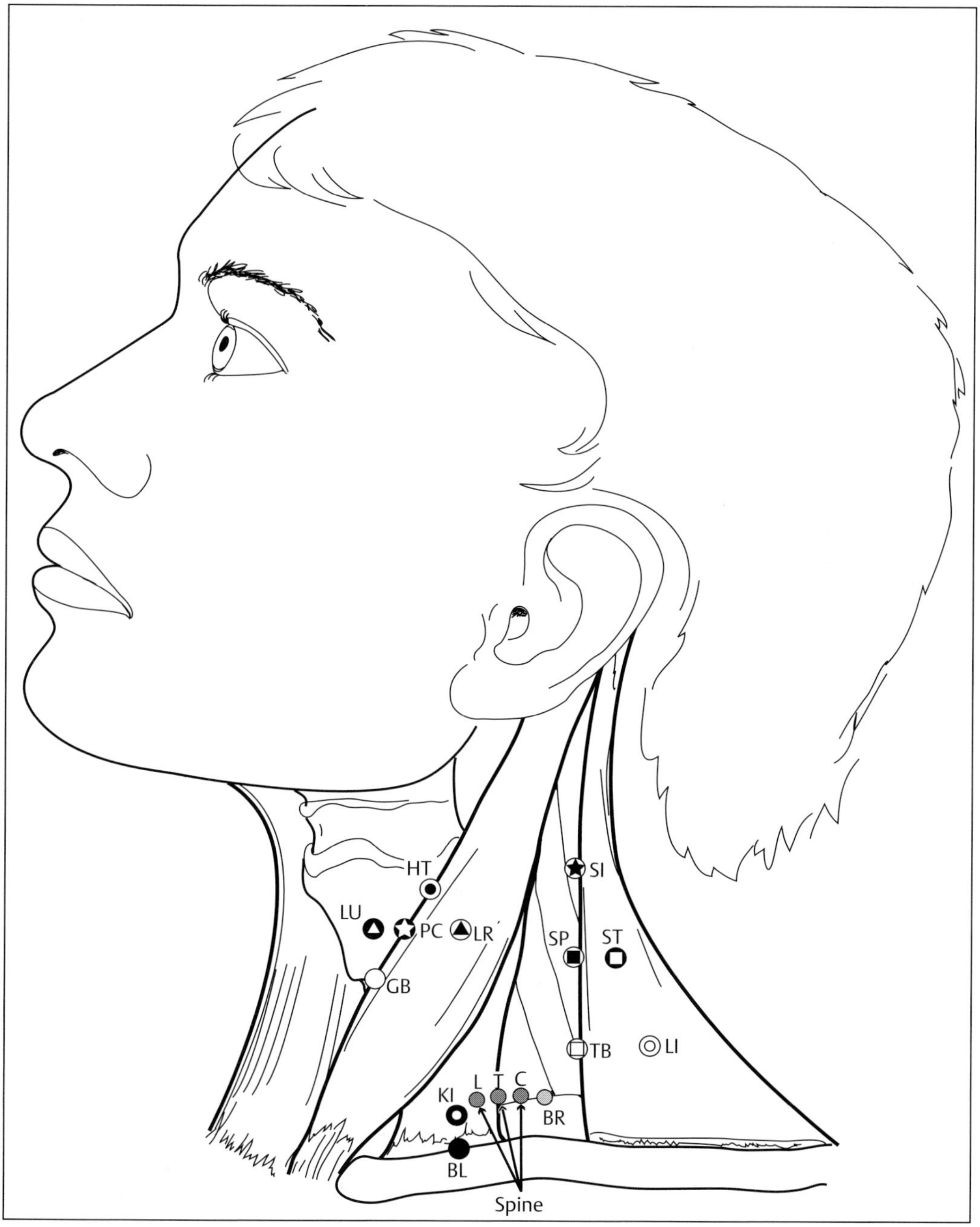

Figure 5–5 YNSA neck diagnosis tender points.

11. From the large intestine (LI), moving medially one thumb breadth underneath the roll of the trapezius muscle is the YNSA neck diagnosis tender point for spleen (SP). If tender, it is positive and needs to be treated.
12. From the spleen (SP), moving superior to SP on top of the trapezius muscle and pressing caudally is the stomach (ST). If tender, it is positive and needs to be treated.
13. From the stomach (ST), moving medially in the hole between the scalenus and trapezius

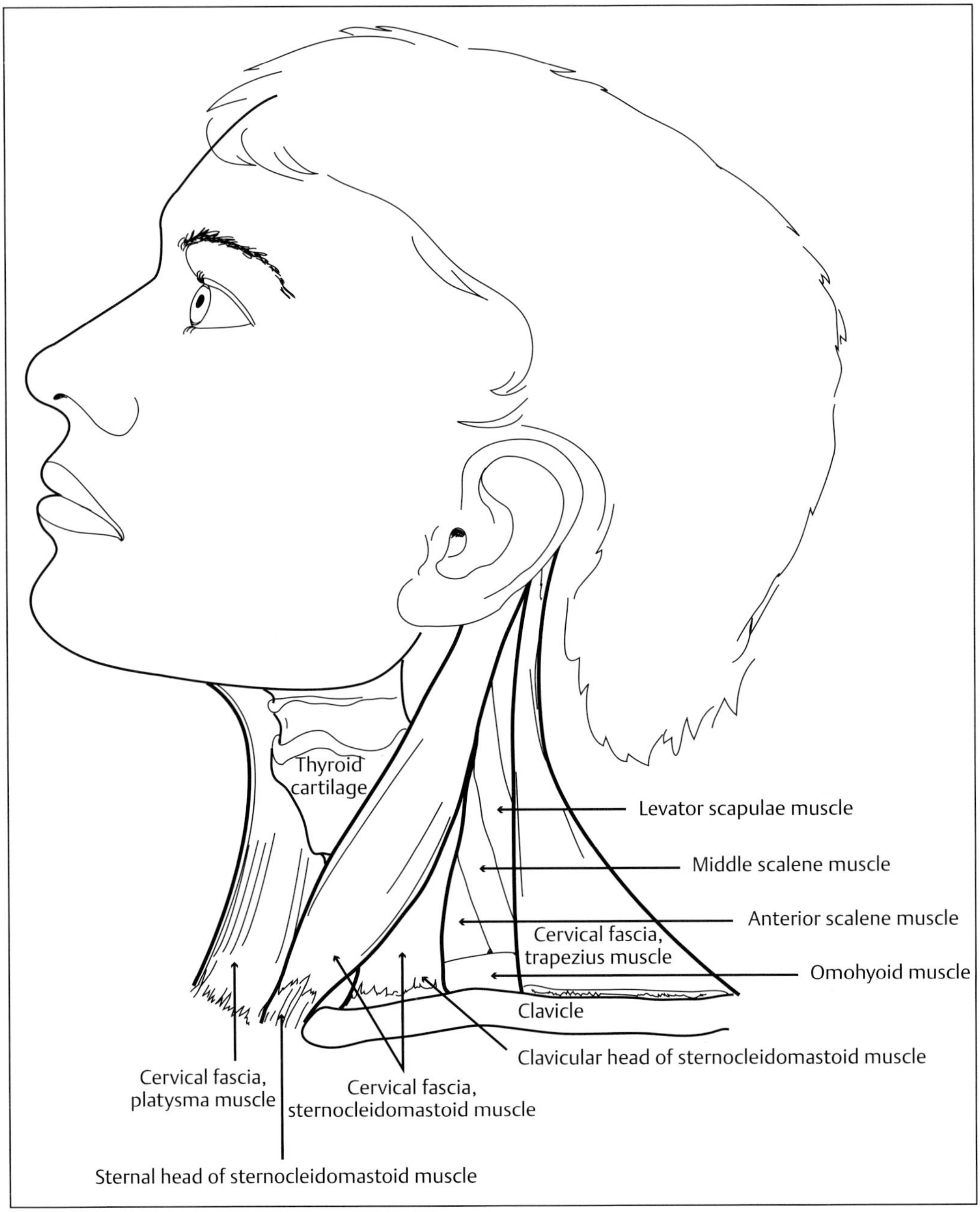

Figure 5–6 Neck anatomy.

muscles, is the small intestine (SI). Press posteriorly to elicit tenderness. If tender, it is positive and needs to be treated.

14. From the small intestine (SI), removing one's thrumb from the trapezius muscle and then placing it next to the thyroid cartilage with the thumbnail medial and pressing posteriorly along the cartilage is the lung (LU). If tender, it is positive and needs to be treated.

YNSA Abdominal Diagnosis

Procedure

YNSA abdominal diagnosis is used to help determine which Ypsilon points to treat; it is also used similarly to YNSA neck diagnosis points. YNSA abdominal diagnosis is used if the neck diagnosis method is not possible or results are indeterminate. Its uniqueness is that the cerebrum, basal ganglia, and cerebellum each have diagnostic tender points. There are six Basic spine points and 12 Ypsilon points related to abdominal zones that, when dysfunctional and then palpated, elicit tension and tenderness.

Method

1. Have the patient supine upon the examination table with the abdomen exposed for palpation.
2. Start in a systematic way to examine the abdomen; see **Figure 5–7** for an anatomical guide. Begin with the brain point group M-1, go to M-2, then to M-3, left and then right. M-1 is just inferior to the xiphoid process in the midline. M-2 is located one finger breadth inferior and lateral to M-1. M-3 is located one finger breadth superior to M-2 and just lateral to M-1. This is where the rib cage joins the sternum. **Figure 5–8** illustrates where each point is found in the abdominal area.
3. Next move over down the abdominal rectus raphe to examine the heart, pericardium, stomach, triple burner, and bladder.
4. Move to the left and begin palpating spleen, liver, large intestine, and left kidney.
5. Then move to the right, starting with the gall bladder, lung, small intestine, and right kidney.
6. For the spine, palpate in the rectus abdominus muscle along the stomach channel line or ~1 cun lateral to the midline.
7. The cervical spine is lateral to the heart, pericardium, and stomach abdominal tender points. Cervical vertebra 1 is most superior and cervical vertebra 7 is the most inferior of the entire 3 cun length of the cervical abdominal tender point.
8. The thoracic spine is lateral to the umbilicus. Thoracic vertebra 1 is ~1.5 cun superior to the umbilicus. Thoracic vertebra 12 is 1.5 cun inferior to the umbilicus, and the rest of the vertebrae are representatively lined up proportionately in order.
9. Lumbar spine is lateral to the triple burner and bladder. Lumbar vertebra 1 is ~2 cun inferior to the umbilicus, and the rest of the lumbar vertebrae follow along in order.

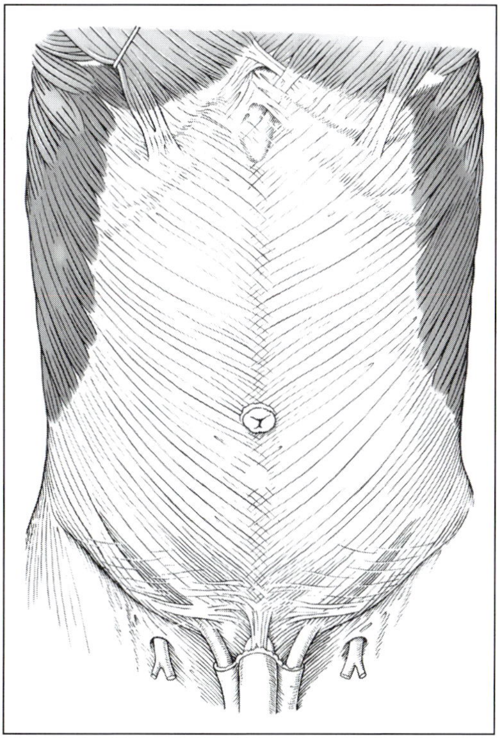

Figure 5–7 Abdominal wall from front: external abdominal oblique (from Werner Platzer, *Color Atlas of Human Anatomy, Vol. 1: Locomotor System*. 5th edition. Thieme: Stuttgart–New York; 2009).

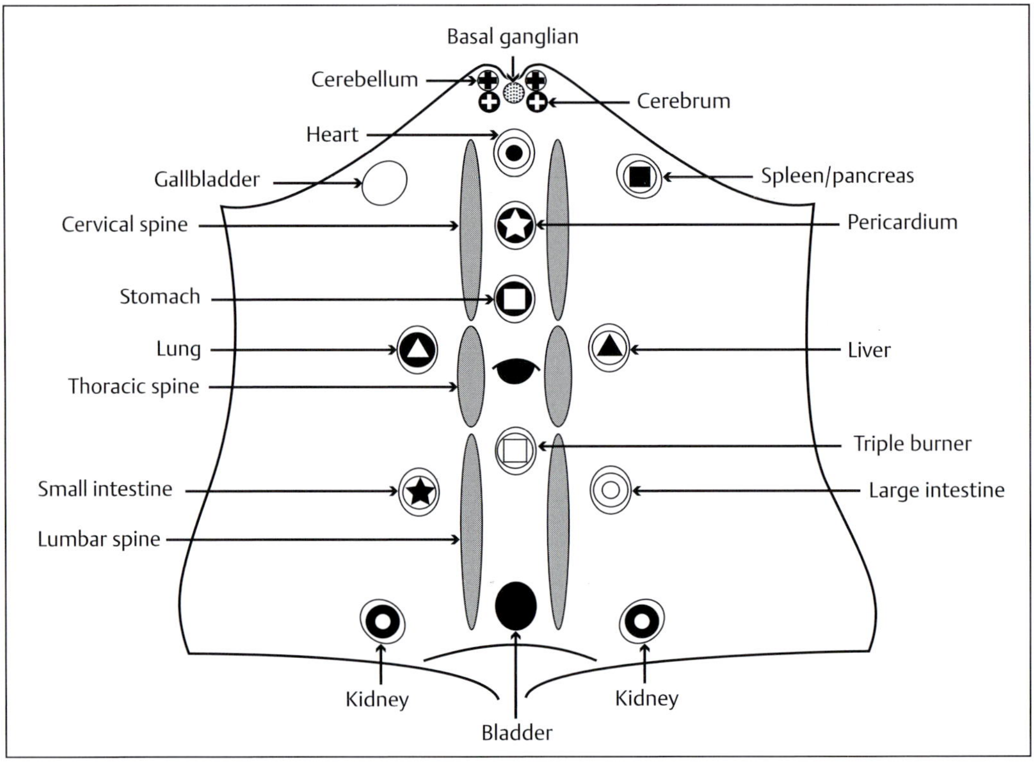

Figure 5–8 YNSA abdominal points.

Pulse Diagnosis

TCM and Five Phase practitioners all use the radial pulse to diagnose the condition of the patient. This is done with the patient seated or lying on a table with the radial artery at or below the heart's height in a sitting or resting position. The hand should never be above the patient's heart. When taking a pulse, three fingers should be used; the index, middle, and ring fingers. With the index finger placed closest to the wrist (inch), the middle finger placed over the styloid process of the radius (bar), and the ring finger placed next to it (cubit) at the most proximal position. This is best done with the practitioner standing, facing the patient, holding the patient's right hand with the practitioner's right hand and the pulse being taken with the left hand. The converse is true for the other side.

At first, three positions are palpated simultaneously; initially lightly, then with medium pressure, and then even more strongly. After this, each position is checked separately and different systems are used whereby the pulse is identified with certain organs, see **Table 5–1**. The system that the author uses is that of the Five Phase system where the left distal (inch) deep pulse relates to the heart, and the superficial pulse relates to the small intestine. The left middle (bar) position deep pulse relates to the liver, and the superficial pulse relates to the gall bladder. The left proximal (cubit) position deep pulse relates to the kidney,

Table 5–1 Five phases zang fu organ pulses

Left			Right	
		Distal		
SI	HT		LU	LI
GB	LR		SP	ST
BL	KI		PC	TB
		Proximal		

and the superficial pulse relates to the bladder. The right radial pulse distal (inch) deep pulse relates to the lung, and the superficial relates to the large intestine. The right middle (bar) position deep pulse relates to the spleen, and the superficial pulse relates to the stomach. The right proximal (cubit) deep pulse relates to the pericardium and the superficial pulse the triple burner.

Using Professor Worsley's Five Phase system of pulse taking and recording, one is concerned with balance between the channels and recording the volume of the pulses. The volumes all relate to what the practitioner would regard as normal for the individual where normal is a check or zero for the ideal pulse volume for that patient's size and state of health. By determining the differences between the six pulses in each wrist, one is able to classify them from a +3 to a –3. Pulses that are found at the three deep levels are compared with each other to determine if one is stronger or weaker than the others. A numerical rating of +3 or –3 is equated to those pulses. If they are all moderate and equal in volume and force, then all three would receive a check or zero. Then the three superficial pulses would be compared with each other in a similar manner. This would be done on both the left and right radial pulses.

Different schools of TCM name different pathological pulses. These schools have a name for 17, 27, 28, and even as many as 32 different pulse types.[2] Some types are very rare and appear only in the late stages of terminal diseases. Others vary only slightly from each other and require considerable experience to determine. The TCM basic quality of pulses includes the following parameters: depth, pace, length, and quality. Under depth, there are two types – floating and submerged. The floating pulse is distinct when the skin is barely touched by the fingertips but fades under greater pressure. This floating pulse is associated with exterior conditions. A submerged pulse is only distinct upon application of considerable pressure and signifies the disorder has advanced to the interior stage.

The pace of a pulse can be described as quick or slow. A quick pulse is six or more beats per breath and signifies heat. A slow pulse is three or fewer beats per breath and signifies cold. The length of the pulse is another important characteristic that can be either long or short. A long pulse can be felt from the proximal portion to below the distal portion. In a healthy person, it represents a robust condition and in an ill person it represents an advanced disease. A short pulse can only be discerned in the middle position and it signifies insufficiency of blood and *qi*.

The two main pulse types for strength are weak and strong. When the pulse feels weak and hardly presses back at the practitioner's fingers, it signifies vacuity in either *qi* or blood. A strong pulse responds strongly to the touch and signifies the presence of repletion in a sick person and a good condition in a healthy person.

The most difficult aspect to ascertain in pulse is the quality. This characteristic includes texture, smoothness, and regularity of the pulse wave.

Some of the diagnostic categories include slippery. A slippery pulse can be definitely discerned but the boundaries are indistinct and as if feeling a ball through a layer of highly viscous liquid. A slippery pulse indicates dampness or phlegm. A rough pulse feels choppy as if waves of the pulse are irregular and signifies congealed blood, stagnant *qi*, or deficient blood. A wiry pulse has a feeling that is long and taut like a violin or guitar string. It is a strong pulse that pushes back and appears in liver disease. A tight pulse feels like a clothesline, much fuller than a wiry pulse; the waves are short and follow each other closely. A huge pulse can be felt at all levels and is slightly stronger on top and at the beginning of the waves. It signifies repletion heat. A fine pulse is small and thin and signifies insufficiency of blood and yin. An irregular pulse has three types all of which signify disorders of heart *qi*. Hasty is fast with irregular pauses and shows repletion heart yang or congested *qi*. A knotted, irregular pulse is slow with irregular pauses and signifies obstruction of blood in the heart or phlegm in the pericardium. An intermittent pulse is systematic but pauses abnormally. This pulse signifies an exhausted condition in the organs. All three pulses are very dangerous signs when they appear in a sick individual. They can appear in a relatively healthy person during periods of mental or emotional strain.

By taking a patient's pulse before YNSA treatment and then after YNSA treatment, one is able to ascertain the effectiveness of that treatment. The goal of the YNSA treatment is to have no more YNSA neck diagnosis or abdominal diagnosis tender points and to have balanced radial pulses; thus one is assured of effective treatment restoring balance and harmony.

Summary

YNSA neck diagnostic techniques are unique, specific, quick, and effective. Abdominal Oriental medicine diagnosis is augmented with YNSA specific points. Oriental medicine, either TCM or Five Phase, pulse diagnoses correlate well with YNSA, but is not required; however, it may be used as an adjunct to YNSA neck diagnosis.

蒙 ䷃ 蒙 ***Méng***

**Childhood—Mountain Above,
Water Below**

*"A Spring flows out of a mountain.
The symbol of an unenlightened ignorant.
In correspondence with this,
The superior person makes every effort
To cultivate virtue with resolute deeds."*[3]

*"Sequence of the Gua: Zhun denotes what has just been born. What has just been born is in its childhood. Thus, after Beginning, Childhood follows.
Decision
Childhood.
Prosperous and smooth.
It is not I who seek the ignorant,
The ignorant seeks me.
On the first divination, I give light.
Repeating again is contemptuous.
Being contemptuous, I give
no more instruction.
Favorable to be steadfast and upright."*[4]

References

Acupoint schema and charts are found on page 144 f.

1. Ming-Dao D. Scholar Warrior: An Introduction to the Tao in Everyday Life. San Francisco: Harper Collins; 1990: 191
2. Kaptchuk TJ. The Web That Has No Weaver: Understanding Chinese Medicine. Chicago: McGraw-Hill; 2000: 299–320
3. Huang A. The Complete I Ching. Rochester, VT: Inner Traditions; 1998: 68
4. Huang A. The Complete I Ching. Rochester, VT: Inner Traditions; 1998: 67

6

YNSA Basic Points

"Those who are well informed of heaven must be able to make corroboration [of their knowledge] in terms of humanity. There is a number 12 [for instance, months] in relation to heaven. [Therefore,] human beings have 12 channels to correspond to it. Heaven is divided into 365 degrees, and humans correspond to it with [as many] qi *points."*[1]

"You can only go halfway into the darkest forest; then you are coming out the other side." – Chinese Proverb

YNSA Basic points. These are the first points used to treat a myriad of diseases based on anatomical pathological correlates and positive YNSA Neck Diagnosis findings.

YNSA Basic points. The first points discovered by Dr. Toshikatsu Yamamoto.

YNSA Basic points. Found in all four quadrants of the scalp.

YNSA Basic points. Some points are lines of points.

YNSA Basic Points

The YNSA Basic points are scalp points that are all ipsilaterally, anatomically correlated. The points were originally named as Dr. Yamamoto discovered them through trial and error as patients present themselves to him in the hospital and clinic. The author further expanded on points that were found to be repeatedly relevant. The Basic points are most frequently used to treat pain in an anatomical area; they are also used to treat disease and dysfunction associated with that particular body part.

The Basic points are found in the YIN and YANG halves of the scalp and are more medial than lateral. There are 23 Basic points found in YIN and 23 Basic points found in YANG. Of the 23 Basic points, there are five Basic points that have subdivisions that are related to individual units, vertebral units, individual vertebrae, and/or parts of the appendicular system. The Basic points that are lines associated with subdivisions of vertebral units are A-1–7 cervical (e.g., A-2 means second cervical vertebra and its related structures, including the spinal nerve root), D-1–6 lumbar (e.g., D-1 means lumbar 1, D-6 means sacrum), E-1–12 thoracic, C-1 upper extremity, and C-2 lower extremity. There are three additional lines that are related to the central nervous system; M-1 represents the basal ganglia and limbic system, M-2 represents the cranial nerves I-XII and the cerebrum, M-3 represents the cerebellum. All the other Basic points are just that—individual points on the scalp. There are 15 individual Basic points in the YIN, front half of the head, and 15 individual Basic points in the YANG, back half of the head. The YIN and YANG Basic points are mirror representations of each other. The individual Basic points are: B-1 shoulder, B-2 foot, D lumbar spine, F sciatic nerve, G-1 medial knee, G-2 patella, G-3 lateral knee, H lumbar spine, I lumbar spine, J foot, K lumbar spine, and the four sensory organ points, which are named after the sensory organs, S-1 eye, S-2 nose, S-3 mouth, and S-4 ear, see **Figures 1–3 and 1–4** in Chapter 1.

For example, if one has neck pain, the A point relates to cervical spine anatomy, which includes bone, cartilage, blood, lymph, nerves, and their neurological functions. Once the diagnosis is made for the pathology, dysfunction, or pain and a determination is made that the patient would benefit from YNSA, the next step is to follow the first, second, third procedures shown in **Figure 5–1** in Chapter 5, and the Basic Point Diagnosis. The first step is to determine which side to treat, left or right. The answer is ipsilateral to the problem. The second procedure is to determine which quadrant to treat, either YIN or YANG. From that determination, one advances to the third procedure and decides which phase of YIN or YANG is to be treated; for example, Yin of YIN or Yang of YIN. The next problem is to find the YNSA Basic point followed by the YNSA Ypsilon point; this can be difficult at first. The Basic and Ypsilon points are always little ridges or mountains in the scalp as you palpate the skull. This psychomotor skill, as well as the needling technique that follows, is best learned one-on-one with an instructor. The companion DVD provides a demonstration of this technique for one to model.

YNSA Basic Point Protocol

Always treat the anatomical correlate ipsilateral to the pain, dysfunction, disease, or tender LI-4 *he gu*.

Use neck diagnosis to confirm the need for treatment. Retest neck diagnosis after needle placement in the scalp to ascertain correct needle placement.

1. Palpate the LI-4, *he gu*, point to determine which side is most tender. If one can not tell the difference with the patient's help, then palpate both left and right LR (liver) neck diagnostic points simultaneously, to see which one is most tender. If one still can not tell which is most tender, then go to the KI (kidney) neck diagnostic point, palpating left and right simultaneously to see which one is tender.
2. Palpate the LR (liver) YNSA neck diagnosis point on the tender side to determine if the sternocleidomastoid muscle (SCM) is hard or soft. If the SCM is soft, treat in YANG. If the SCM is firm, treat in YIN. Furthermore, if the SCM is hard/firm, treat in Yin of YIN. If the SCM is superficial soft/hard underneath, treat in Yang of YIN. If the SCM is firm/soft underneath, treat in Yin of YANG. If the SCM is soft/soft, treat in Yang of YANG. More than 90% of

the time, it is hard, so treat in the YIN phase. Less than 10% of the time, it is soft and to be treated in the YANG phase.
3. YNSA Basic point neck diagnosis is done by palpating the lumbar, thoracic, cervical, and brain points. Tenderness indicates a positive finding and need for YNSA treatment of the correct Basic point. Follow the procedure in **Figure 5–2** in Chapter 5.

Scalp and Body Measurements

All descriptions are given in Chinese acupuncture measurements, cun, because in practice it is easier to use finger measurements in determining point locations as opposed to a metric ruler. A cun is, specifically a patient's one body inch, see **Figures 6–1 and 6–2**, the anatomical measurement of the patient's middle phalanx of the index finger or the width of the patient's thumb. By correlating your index finger middle phalanx with that of your patient, you will be using the correct measurement on various size patients, see **Figures 6–3, 6–4, and 6–5.** One index finger breadth is ~0.5 cun. Other measurements will be noted in millimeters (mm) or centimeters (cm).

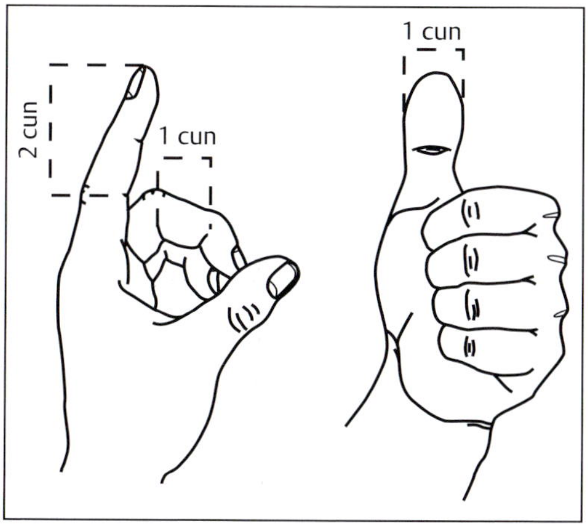

Figure 6–1 1 and 2 cun measurements.

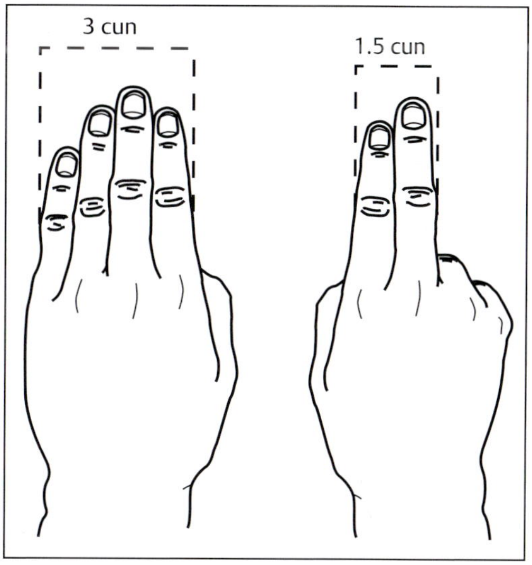

Figure 6–2 1.5 and 3 cun measurements.

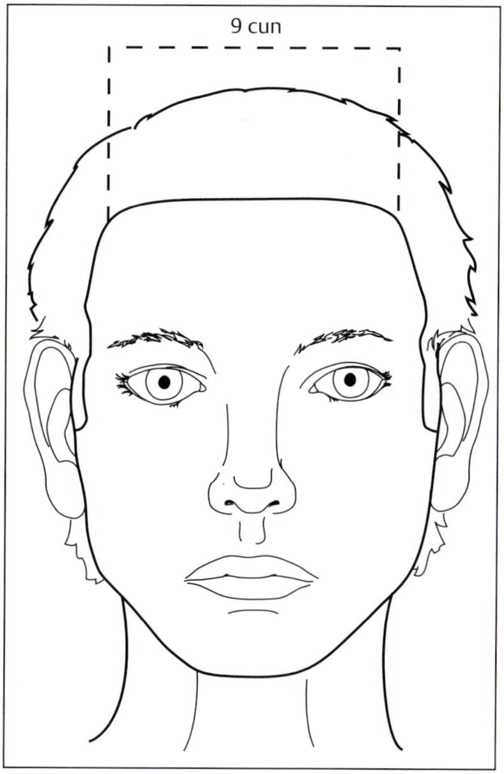

Figure 6–3 Forehead cun measurement.

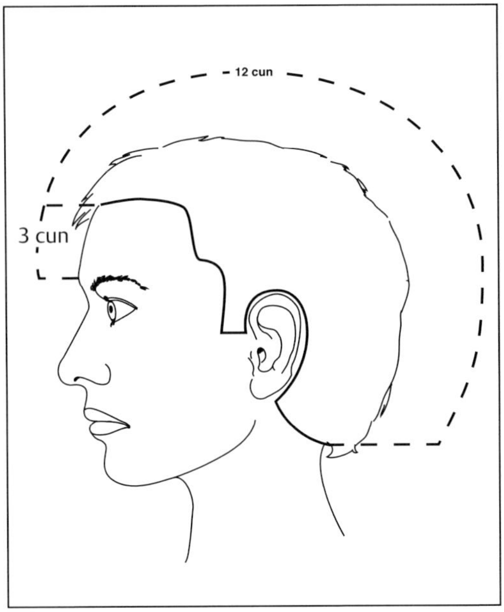

Figure 6–4 Lateral head cun measurement.

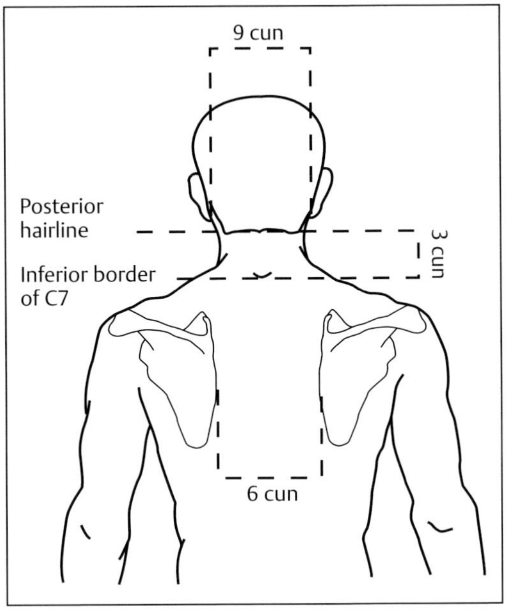

Figure 6–5 Back of head cun measurement.

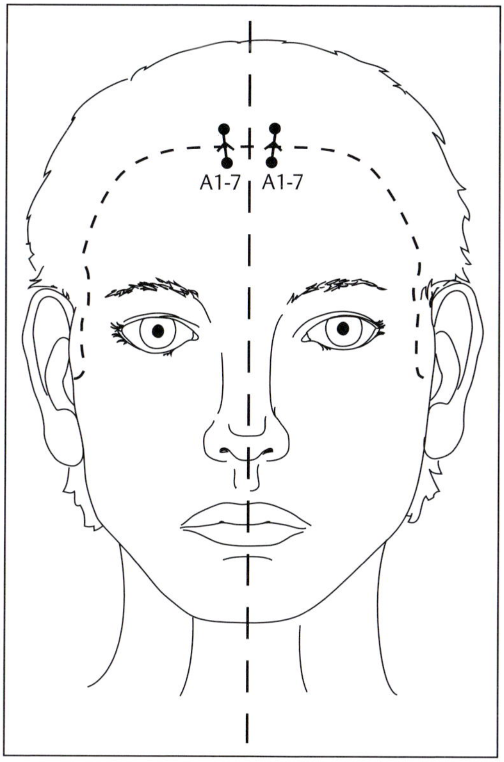

Figure 6–6 Basic point A-1–7 Yin.

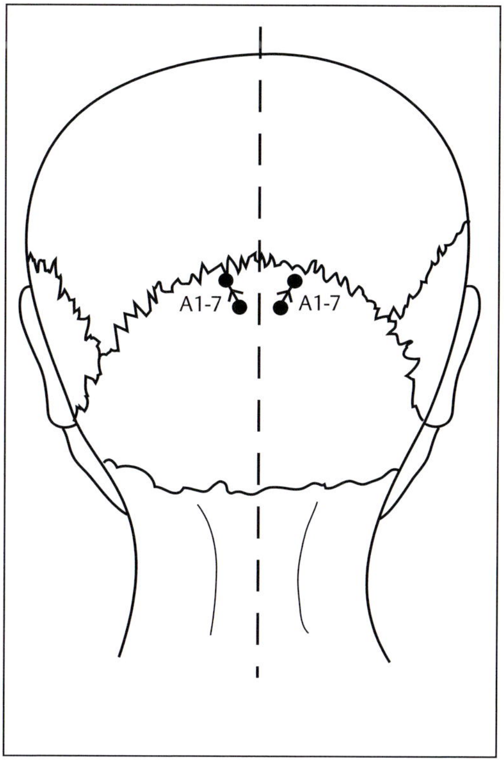

Figure 6–7 Basic point A-1–7 Yang.

YNSA Somatotope of the Scalp: Basic Points

Points A-1–7

Anatomical Correlates

Ipsilateral: Cervical spine vertebrae C1–7, C1–8 nerve motor and sensory distribution affects and effects, C1–7 discs and fascia, cervical musculature, and soft tissue structures of the neck.

Location

A point is a line of points representing the entire cervical spine.

Yin of YIN: At the hairline, 0.5 cun lateral to the metopic suture of the frontal bone, see **Figure 6–6**. In Yin of YIN, cervical nerve root 3 (C3) is located at the hairline, cervical nerve 1 root (C1) is located a few millimeters below the hairline, whereas C8, the eighth cervical nerve root, is located more centrally (posterior) along the line of the A points, ~30 mm posterior to the hairline.

Yin of YANG: At the superior nuchal line ~0.5 cun lateral to midline of the occipital bone, see **Figure 6–7**. C1 is located caudal/inferior. C8 is located more centrally (anterior) along the A line point ~40 mm anterior to the superior nuchal line toward the lambdoidal suture.

Technique

Palpate the slight ridge or contraction of the areola tissue of the scalp. Piqué subcutaneously at a 70 degree angle over the representative cervical correlate. If treating more than one vertebra correlate, change the needle angle to 15 degrees, then thread the needle along the ridge.

Purpose and Use

This anatomical point is especially useful when a positive neck diagnosis is made, but may be used based on known anatomical relationships to the

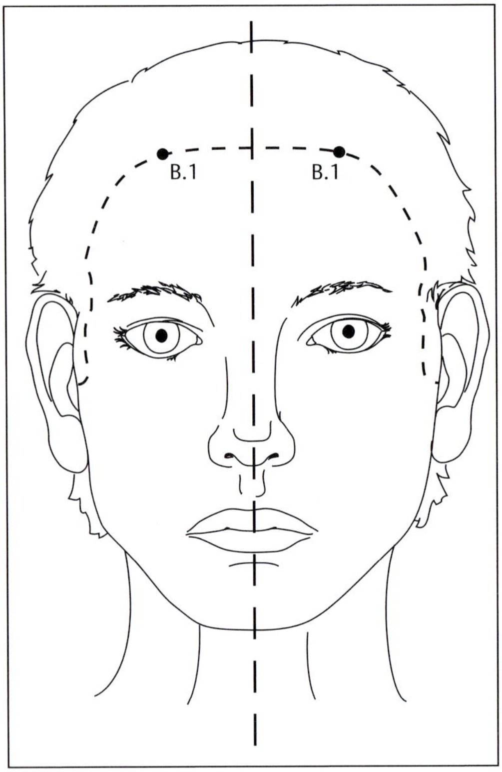

Figure 6–8 Basic point B-1 Yin.

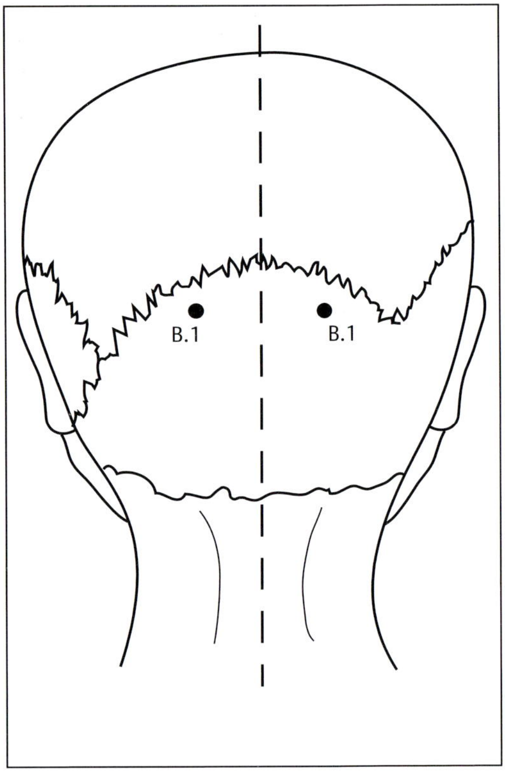

Figure 6–9 Basic point B-1 Yang.

patient's disease, dysfunction, and/or point tenderness. This point is effective for cervical pain and dysfunction: cervicalgia, myositis, cervical radiculopathy, tension cephalgia, migraine, acceleration/deceleration syndrome/whiplash, vertigo, neuritis, neuralgia, cerebral disturbances, facial paralysis, toothache, and vegetative disturbances.

Point B-1

Anatomical Correlate

Ipsilateral: Acromial-clavicular joint and glenohumeral joint and related soft tissue structures.

Location

Yin of YIN: At the hairline, 1.2 cun lateral to the metopic suture or 0.7 cun lateral to the line of the A points, see **Figure 6–8**. The point is ~3 mm in length.

Yin of YANG: On the superior nuchal ridge 1.0 cun lateral to the midline of the occiput, see **Figure 6–9**. The point is ~3 mm in length.

Technique

Palpate the slight ridge or contraction of the areola tissue of the scalp.

Piqué subcutaneously at a 70 degree angle over the point.

Purpose and Use

All shoulder joint pain and pathology, including rotator cuff pain, osteoarthritis, hemiplegia, paraplegia, tendonitis, and bursitis

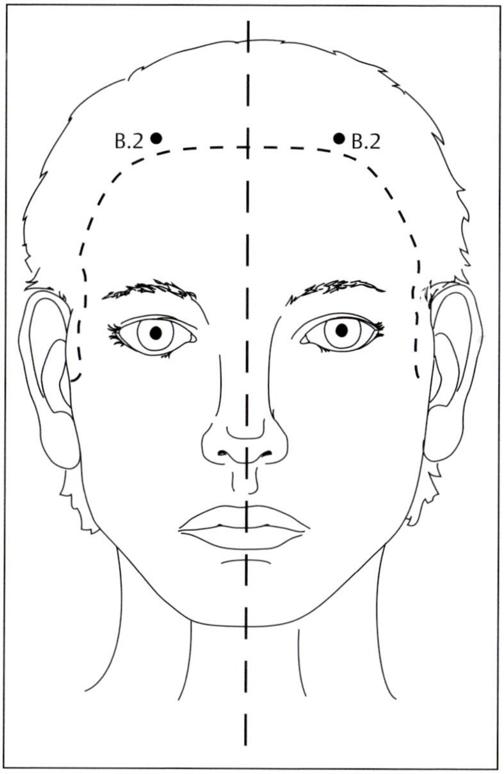

Figure 6–10 Basic point B-2 Yin.

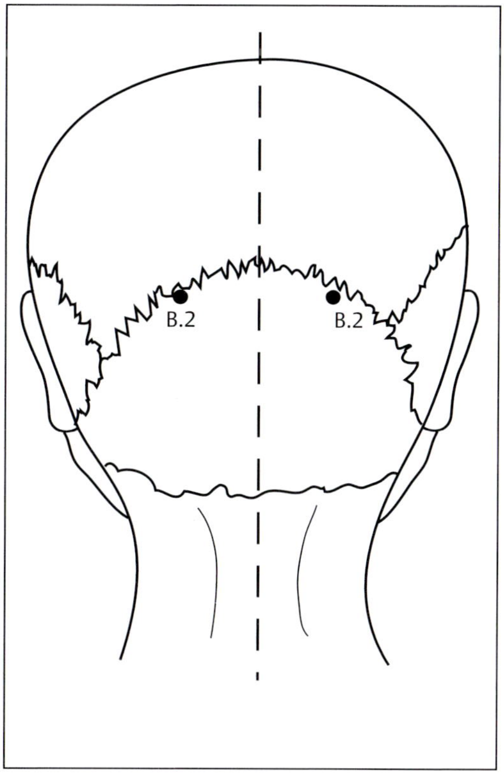

Figure 6–11 Basic point B-2 Yang.

Point B-2

Anatomical Correlate

Ipsilateral: Foot and related soft tissue structures.

Location

Yin of YIN: About 0.5 cun posterior to the hairline 1.2 cun lateral to the metopic suture or 0.7 cun lateral to Point A, see **Figure 6–10**. The point is ~3 mm in length. Yin of YANG: On the lambdoidal suture area 0.25 cun lateral to the line of the A points on the occiput, see **Figure 6–11**. The point is ~3 mm in length.

Technique

Palpate the slight ridge or contraction of the areola tissue of the scalp. Piqué subcutaneously at a 70 degree angle over the point.

Purpose and Use

Foot pain, neuropathy, neuralgia, neuritis, and dysfunction

Point C-1

Anatomical Correlate

Ipsilateral: Entire arm from shoulder to finger joints and related soft tissue structures.

Location

Point C-1 is a line of points representing the entire upper extremity, see **Figure 6–12**.

Yin of YIN: At the hairline 2.0 cun lateral to the metopic suture or 1.5 cun lateral to the line of point A. The line is ~1 cun or ~45 mm in length. The C-1 line takes a 30 degree angle from the hairline toward the nari. The hairline correlates to the shoulder; the elbow is one-third of the way down

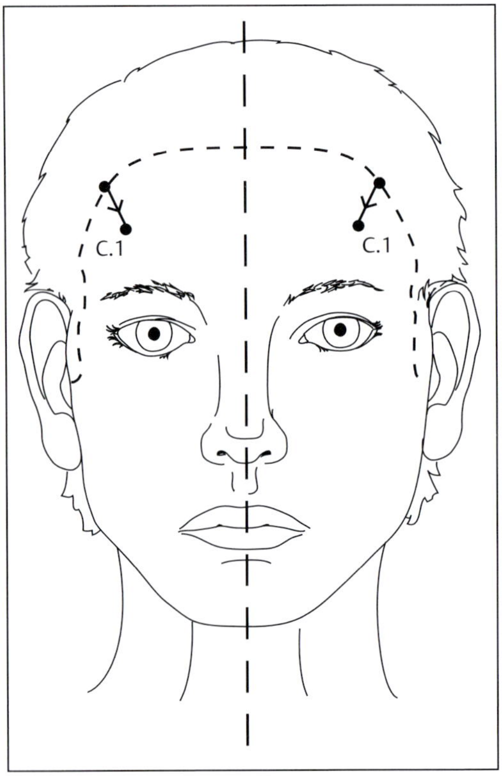

Figure 6–12 Basic point C-1 Yin.

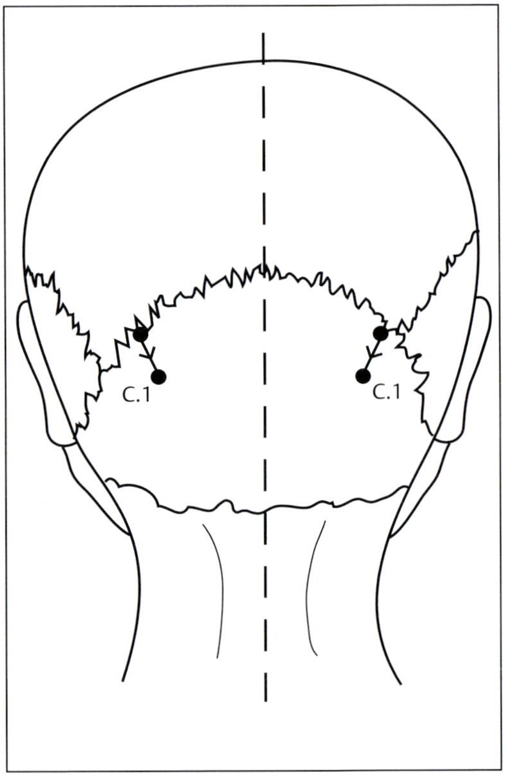

Figure 6–13 Basic point C-1 Yang.

the C-1 line on frontal bone. The wrist and fingers are displayed in supinated position, correlating downward on the frontal bone.

Yin of YANG: On the superior nuchal ridge 1.5 cun lateral to the midline of the occiput, along the lamboidal suture. The line is ~1 cun or ~45 mm in length, see **Figure 6–13**. It is a mirror image of the front Yin of YIN point and runs similarly.

Technique

Palpate the slight ridge or contraction of the areola tissue of the scalp at the hairline. Piqué subcutaneously at a 70 degree angle over the point that correlates to the anatomical part to be treated. Change the angle to 15 degrees to thread the needle along the C-1 line; you may piqué the entire length of the point if needed.

Purpose and Use

All shoulder, arm, and hand pain and dysfunctions. All upper motor and lower motor lesions that affect the shoulder, arm, hand, and fingers: frozen shoulder, and trauma such as dislocation, sprain, fractures, tendonitis, bursitis, rheumatoid arthritis, Parkinson's disease, multiple sclerosis, circulatory disturbances.

Point C-2

Anatomical Correlate

Ipsilateral: Entire leg from hip to toe joints and related soft tissue structures

Location

Point C-2 is a line of points representing the entire lower extremity.

Yin of YIN: At the hairline, 2.0 cun lateral to the metopic suture or 1.5 cun lateral to the line of point A, see **Figures 6–14, 6–15, and 6–16**. The C-2 line takes a 30 degree angle from the hairline toward the nari. The point is ~1 cun or ~45 mm in

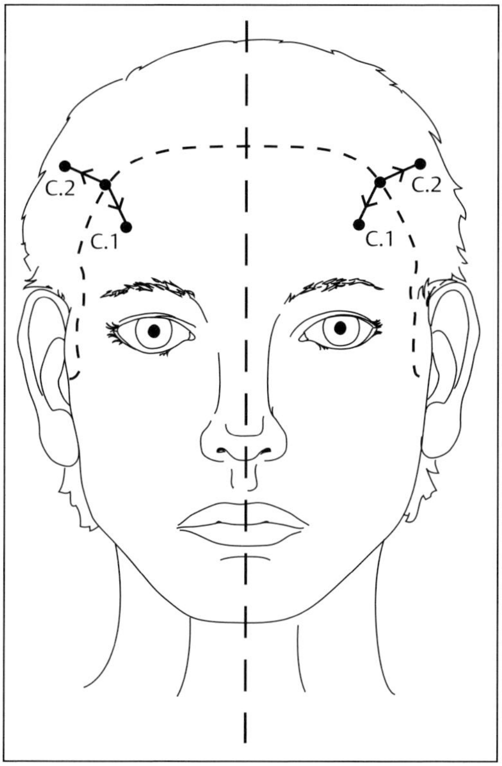

Figure 6–14 Basic point C-1–2 Yin.

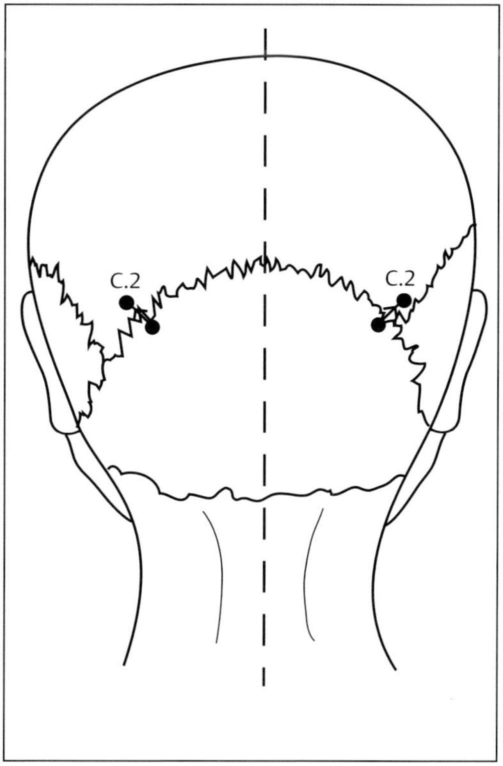

Figure 6–15 Basic point C-2 Yang.

length. The hairline correlates to the hip, the knee is one-third of the way down the line on the frontal bone. The ankle and toes are displayed in an externally rotated position correlated down the line on the frontal bone.

Yin of YANG: On the superior nuchal ridge 1.5 cun lateral to the midline of the occiput.

The point is ~1 cun or ~45 mm in length. It is a mirror image of the front Yin of YIN point and runs similarly.

Technique

Palpate the slight ridge or contraction of the areola tissue of the scalp at the hairline. Piqué subcutaneously at a 70 degree angle over the point that correlates to the anatomical part to be treated. Change the angle to 15 degrees to thread the needle along the C-2 line; you may piqué the entire length of the point with one needle if needed.

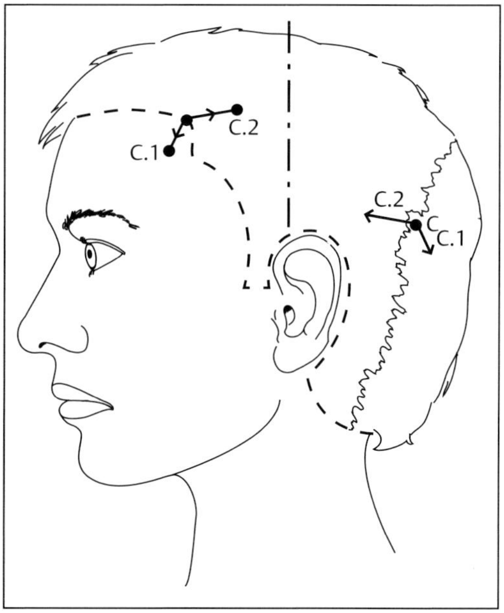

Figure 6–16 Lateral Basic point C-1–2 Yin/Yang.

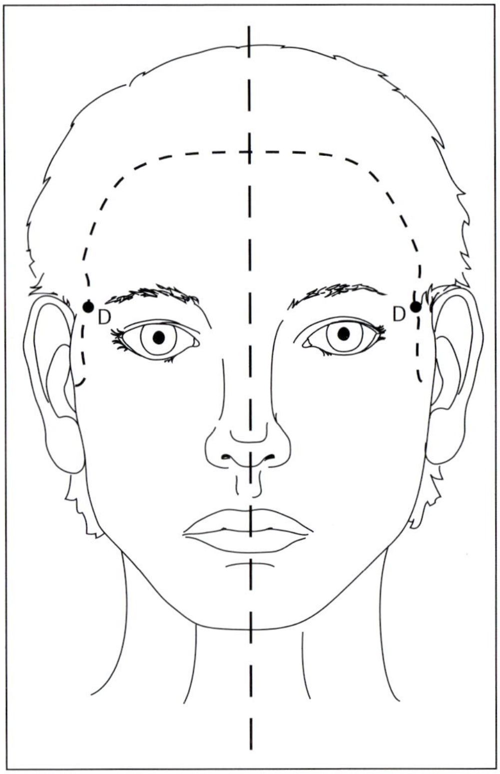

Figure 6–17 Basic point D Yin.

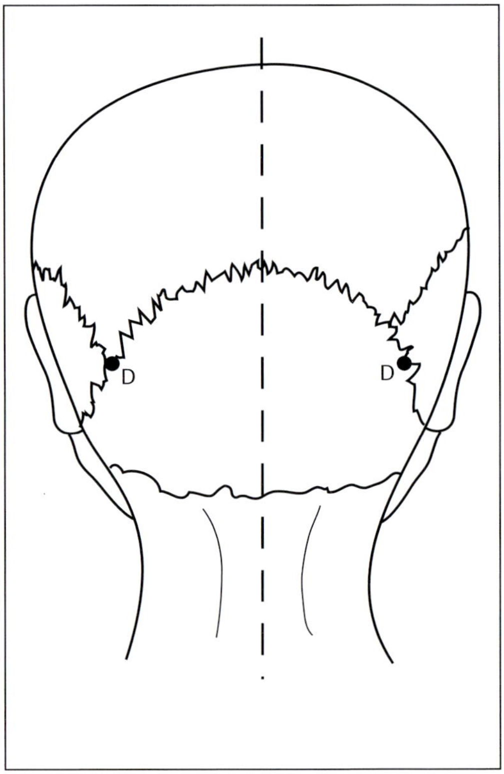

Figure 6–18 Basic point D Yang.

Purpose and Use

All hip, leg, and foot pain and dysfunctions. All upper motor and lower motor lesions that affect the hip, leg, foot, and toes, trauma, dislocation, sprain, fractures, tendonitis, bursitis, bunions, osteoarthritis, rheumatoid arthritis, Parkinson's disease, multiple sclerosis, circulatory disturbances.

Point D

Anatomical Correlate

Ipsilateral: Entire lower extremity and lumbar spine

Location

Yin of YIN: at the edge of the hairline, 0.25 cun superior to the zygomatic process of the temporal bone, see **Figure 6–17**.

Yin of YANG: 1 cun lateral to C-1 along the lambdoidal suture on the occiput. Palpate for a small hill, see **Figure 6–18**.

Technique

Palpate the slight ridge or contraction of the areola tissue of the scalp at the hairline. Piqué subcutaneously at a 70 degree angle over the point.

Purpose and Use

All lower extremity and lumbar spinal joints and related soft tissue pain and dysfunction. All upper motor and lower motor lesions that affect the lower extremity, hip, knee, foot, and toes: sciatica, lumbago, herniated lumbar disc, neuralgia, neuritis, hemiplegia, paraplegia, trauma, dislocation, sprain, fractures, tendonitis, bursitis, rheumatoid arthritis, Parkinson's disease, multiple sclerosis, gout, Raynaud's disease, circulatory disturbances.

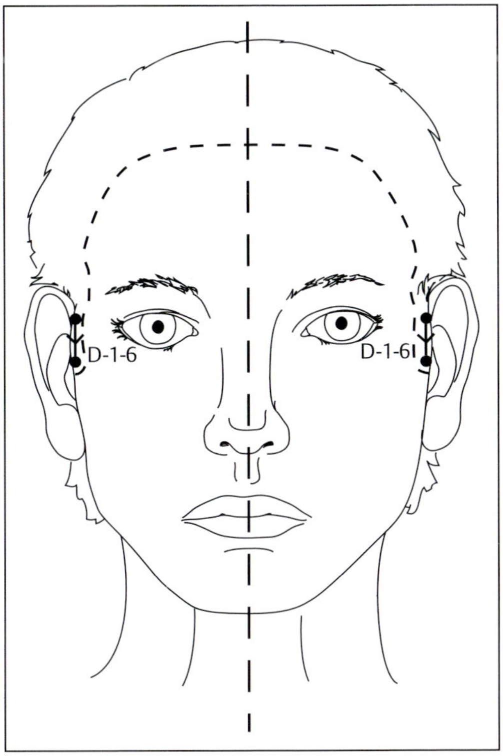

Figure 6–19 Basic point D-1–6 Yin.

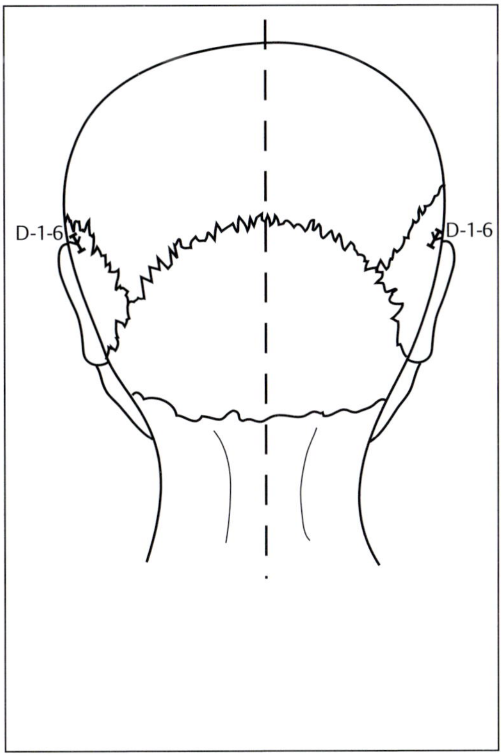

Figure 6–20 Basic point D-1–6 Yang.

Points D-1–6

Anatomical Correlate

Ipsilateral: Entire lumbar spine, soma and neural structures including their related vascular and lymphatic elements. Primarily related to L1–S2 nerve roots and their function. L1 is most superior and coccyx is most caudal in both YIN and YANG quadrants. Lumbar spine vertebrae L1–5 and sacral S1–2 nerve, motor, and sensory distribution affects and effects, L1–5, sacrum, and coccyx, discs, fascia, lumbar musculature, and soft tissue structures of the spine, hips, pelvis, and lower extremity.

Location

Points D-1–6 are a line of points representing all lumbar vertebrae, sacrum and coccyx.

Yin of YIN: at the posterior hairline of the sideburn, 0.5 cun above the zygomatic arch of the temporal bone, in front of the root of the pinna of the ear, see **Figure 6–19**.

Yin of YANG: at the hairline behind the pinna of the ear, 0.5 cun posterior to the root of the pinna of the ear on the temporal bone, see **Figures 6–20 and 6–21**. The point is ~3 mm in length.

Technique

Palpate the area just in front of the root of the ear. There is no ridge or hill. Piqué subcutaneously at a 15 degree angle over the point that correlates with the anatomical part to be treated. You may piqué the entire length of the line with one needle if needed.

Purpose and Use

This anatomical point is especially useful when a positive neck diagnosis is made for lumbar spine, but may be used based on known anatomical relationships to the patient's disease and dysfunction. This point is effective for lumbar pain, dysfunction, and disease, particularly herniated discs.

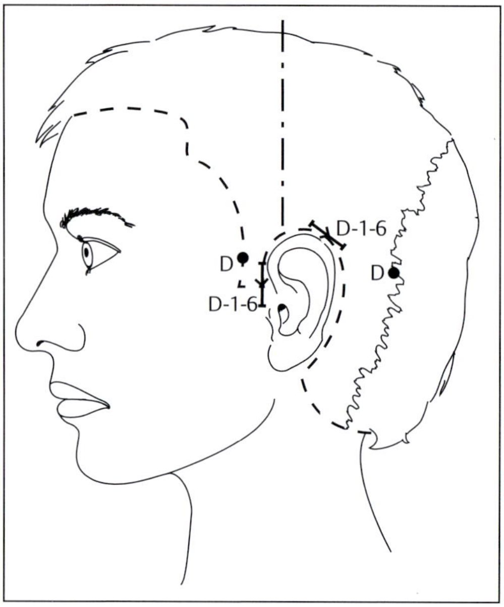

Figure 6–21 Lateral Basic point D and D-1–6 Yin/Yang.

All upper motor and lower motor lesions that affect the lower extremity, hip, knee, foot, and toes: sciatica, lumbago, herniated lumbar disc, neuralgia, neuritis, neuropathy, hemiplegia, paraplegia, trauma, dislocation, sprain, fractures, tendonitis, bursitis, rheumatoid arthritis, Parkinson's disease, ankylosing spondylitis, multiple sclerosis, gout, Raynaud's disease, circulatory disturbances.

Points E-1–12

Anatomical Correlate

Ipsilateral: Entire thoracic spine soma and neural structures including their related vascular and lymphatic elements. E-1, connected to T1, is lateral and most superior, whereas E-12 is most medial and inferior in both YIN and YANG positions. The points on the E line relate to the thoracic spine vertebrae T1–12 nerve, motor, and sensory distribution affects and effects, T1–12 discs and fascia, thoracic musculature and soft tissue structures of the spine, trunk, and rib cage.

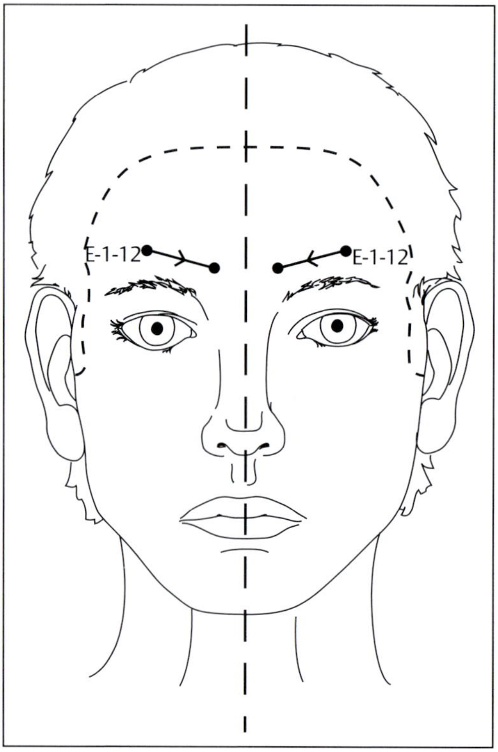

Figure 6–22 Basic point E-1–12 Yin.

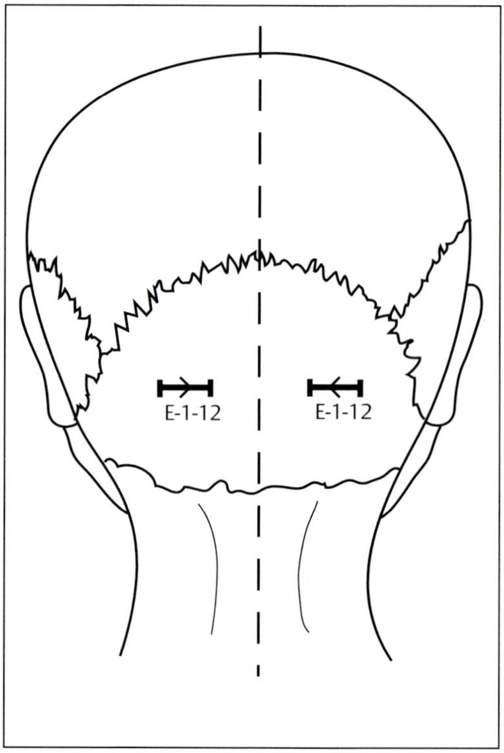

Figure 6–23 Basic point E-1–12 Yang.

Location

Points E-1–12 are a line representing thoracic vertebrae 1–12, similar to D-1–6 representing lumbar vertebrae.

Yin of YIN: located above the eyebrow; T12 starts 0.5 cun lateral to the midline above the supra orbital rim. T1 is located lateral at a 15 degree angle 1.75 to ~2 cun, see **Figure 6–22**.

Yin of YANG: on the occiput under the supraoccipital ridge, T1 is located 1 cun lateral to the midline; points E-1–12 are located moving 1.25 cun superior at a 15 degree angle, see **Figure 6–23**.

Technique

Palpate the area for tenderness. Piqué subcutaneously at a 15 degree angle over the point that correlates with the anatomical part to be treated. You may piqué the entire length of the point line if needed.

Purpose and Use

This anatomical point is especially useful when a positive neck diagnosis is made for thoracic spine, but may be used based on known anatomical relationships to the patient's disease and dysfunction. This point is effective for thoracic pain and dysfunction. All upper and lower motor lesions that affect the trunk, herniated thoracic disc, neuralgia, neuritis, neuropathy, hemiplegia, paraplegia, rib and thoracic trauma, dislocation, sprain, fractures, costochondritis, herpes zoster, angina pectoris, dyspnea, asthma, bronchitis, pneumonia, and circulatory disturbances.

Point F

Anatomical Correlate

Ipsilateral: Sciatic nerve.

Location

Only found in the Yang position. Located on the mastoid process, the most protuberant tender point retroauricularly, see **Figure 6–24**. This point is ~3 mm in length.

Technique

Palpate the highest point, little mountain, or contraction of tissue over the mastoid process. Piqué subcutaneously at a 70 degree angle over the point.

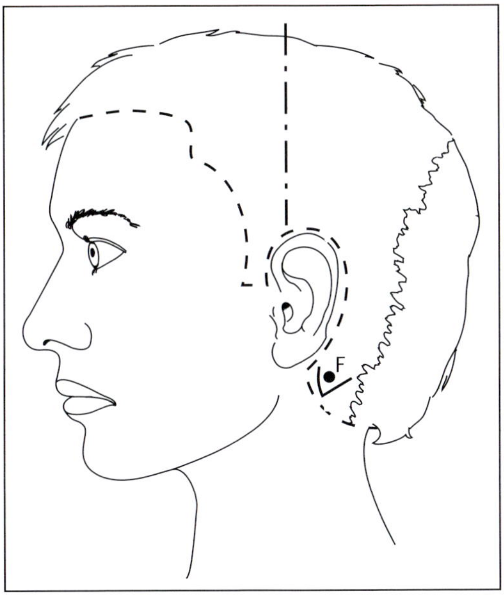

Figure 6–24 Basic point F Lateral.

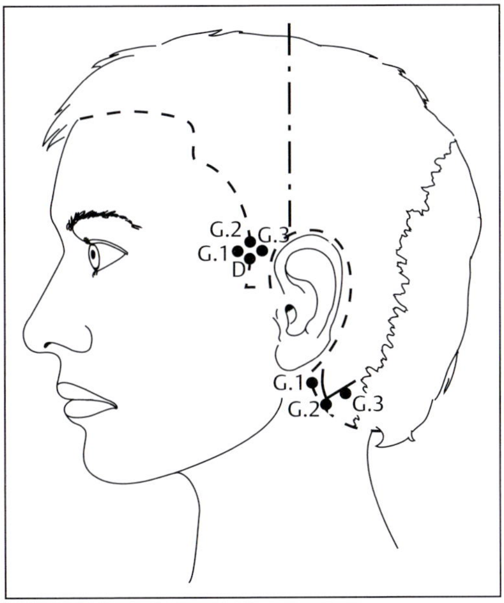

Figure 6–25 Basic point G-1, G-2, and G-3 Lateral.

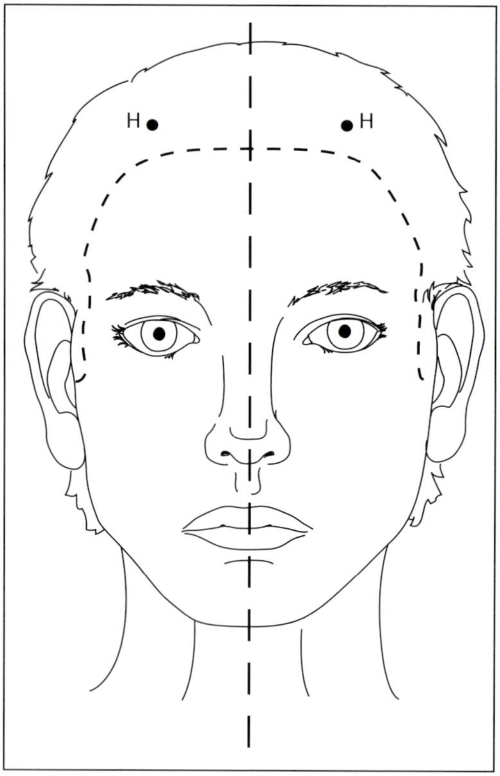

Figure 6–26 Basic point H Yin.

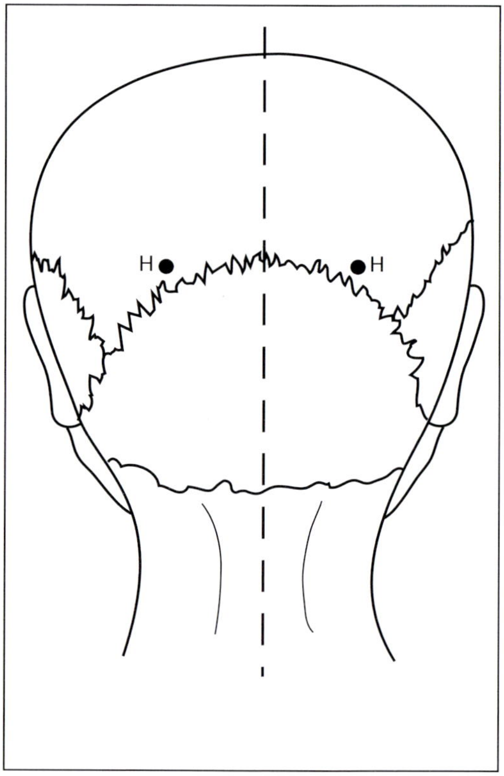

Figure 6–27 Basic point H Yang.

Purpose and Use

This is the principle point for sciatica. Used for sciatica and lumbar radiculopathy.

Points G-1–3

Anatomical Correlate

Ipsilateral: Medial knee is G-1, patella is G-2, and lateral knee is G-3.

Location

Yin of YIN: In a line, G-1 is anterior, G-2 is slightly superior and between G-1 and G-2 G-3 is most posterior. They are ~0.2 cun above points on the D line; see **Figure 6–25**. Each point is ~2 mm in length.

Yin of YANG: On the mastoid process, G-2 is located at the tip of the mastoid at the root of the styloid. G-1 is located 0.5 cun anterior and 0.5 cun superior to G-2. G-3 is located 0.5 cun posterior and 0.5 cun superior to G-2. Each point is ~3 mm in length.

Technique

Palpate the edge of the mastoid process, identify the tip, and then piqué the point needed, either G-1–3 or any of three points individually. The point is usually tender to palpation. Piqué subcutaneously at a 70 degree angle over the point.

Purpose and Use

Knee pain, neuralgia, neuritis, bursitis, meniscus tears, sprains, osteoarthritis, chondromalacia of the patella, fracture, capsular sprain, strains, and somatic dysfunction.

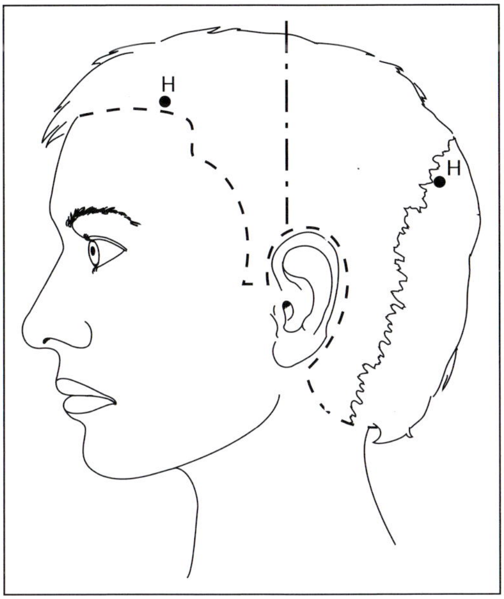

Figure 6–28 Lateral Basic point H Yin/Yang.

Point H

Anatomical Correlate

Ipsilateral: Point H is a supplementary point for lumbar symptomatology. It is not used alone but in conjunction with point D and/or points D-1–6.

Location

Yin of YIN: Caudally ~0.5 cun posterior to B-2. The point is ~3 mm in length, see **Figure 6–26**.

Yin of YANG: Superior ~0.25 cun anterior to B-2. The point is ~3 mm in length, see **Figures 6–27 and 6–28**.

Technique

Palpate the tender high point of the scalp. Piqué subcutaneously at a 70 degree angle over the point.

Purpose and Use

Used in conjunction with basic D and D-1–6 points for unrelenting lumbar symptomatology.

Point I

Anatomical Correlate

Ipsilateral: Point I is a supplementary point for lumbar symptomatology. It is rarely used alone but more commonly in conjunction with point D and/or points D-1–6.

Location

Yin of YIN: Caudally ~1.0 cun behind C-2, see **Figure 6–29**. The point is ~3 mm in length.

Yin of YANG: Superior ~0.5 cun anterior to C-2, see **Figures 6–30 and 6–31**. The point is ~3 mm in length.

Technique

Palpate the tender high point of the scalp. Piqué subcutaneously at a 70 degree angle.

Point J

Anatomical Correlate

Ipsilateral: Point J is a supplementary point for dorsal foot pain. It is rarely used alone but in conjunction with points D and/or C-2 and/or B-2.

Location

Yang of YIN: At the vertex of the head on the parietal bone, 0.5 cun anterior to the transverse line. The point is a little hill, tender to touch, ~3 mm in length, see **Figure 6–32**.

Yang of YANG: At the vertex of the head on the parietal bone, 0.5 cun posterior to the transverse line. The point is a little hill, tender to touch, ~3 mm in length.

Technique

Palpate the tender high point of the scalp. Piqué subcutaneously at a 70 degree angle over the point.

Purpose and Use

Used in conjunction with basic C-2, B-2, and/or points on the D line for dorsal foot pain.

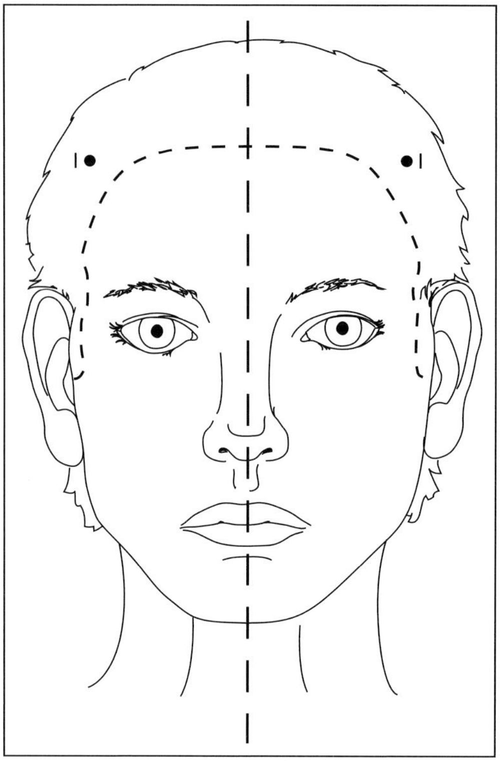

Figure 6–29 Basic point I Yin.

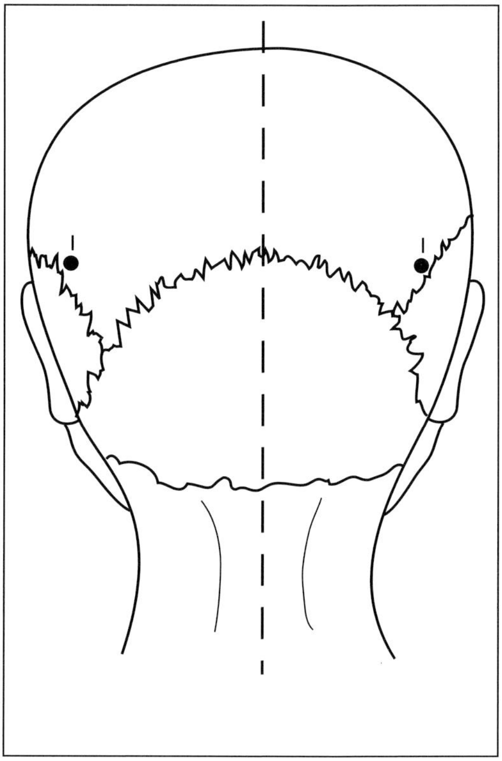

Figure 6–30 Basic point I Yang.

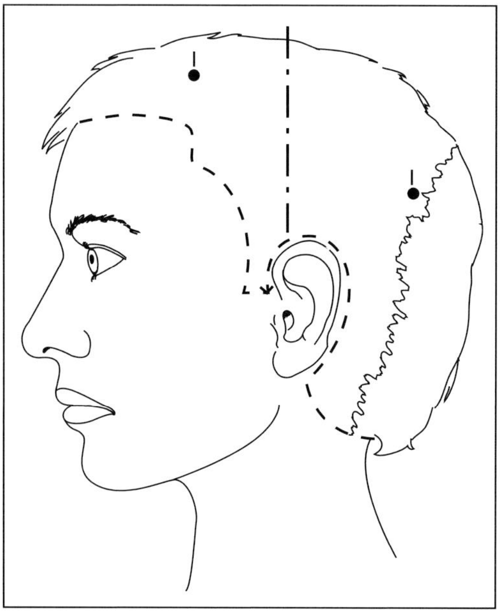

Figure 6–31 Lateral Basic point I Yin/Yang.

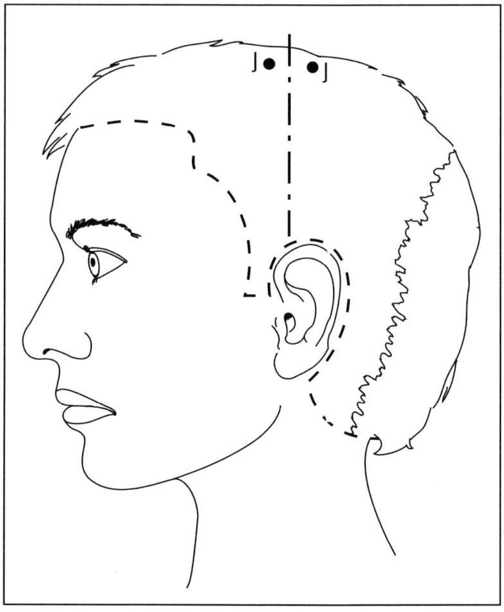

Figure 6–32 Basic point J Yin/Yang.

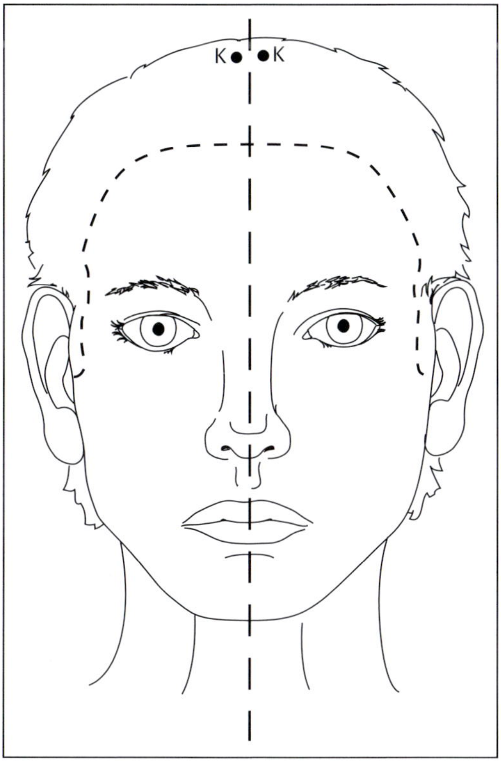

Figure 6–33 Basic point K Yin.

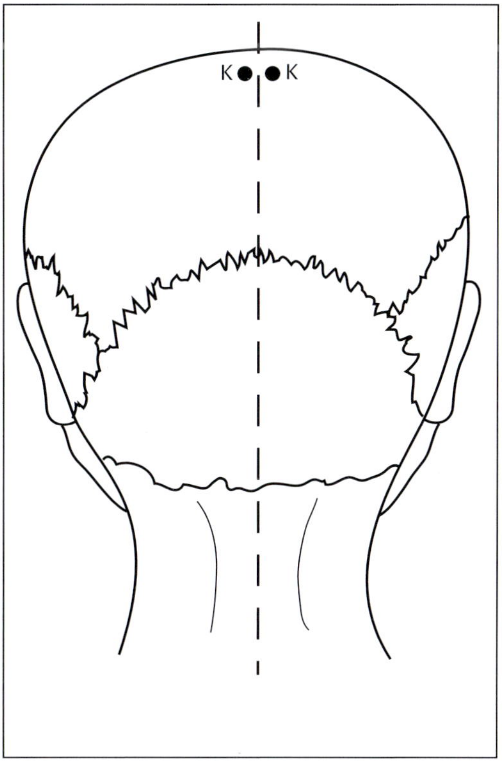

Figure 6–34 Basic point K Yang.

Point K

Anatomical Correlate

Ipsilateral: Point K is a supplementary point for lumbar symptomatology particularly herniated disc. It is rarely used alone but in conjunction with D and/or C-2 and/or points D-1–6.

Location

Yang of YIN: At the vertex of the head on the parietal bone 1 cun anterior to the transverse line. The point is a little hill, tender to touch, ~3 mm in length, see **Figure 6–33**.

Yang of YANG: At the vertex of the head on the parietal bone 1.0 cun posterior to the transverse line, see **Figure 6–34**. The point is a little hill, tender to touch, ~3 mm in length.

Technique

Palpate the tender high point of the scalp. Piqué subcutaneously at a 70 degree angle over the point.

Purpose and Use

This point is used in conjunction with basic D and D-1–6 points for unrelenting lumbar pain and herniated disc.

Points M-1, M-2, and M-3

Anatomical Correlates

Ipsilateral: Points M-1, M-2, and M-3 are named for midline brain points. The basal ganglion is M-1, cranial nerves I-XII and cerebrum are M-2, and cerebellum is M-3.

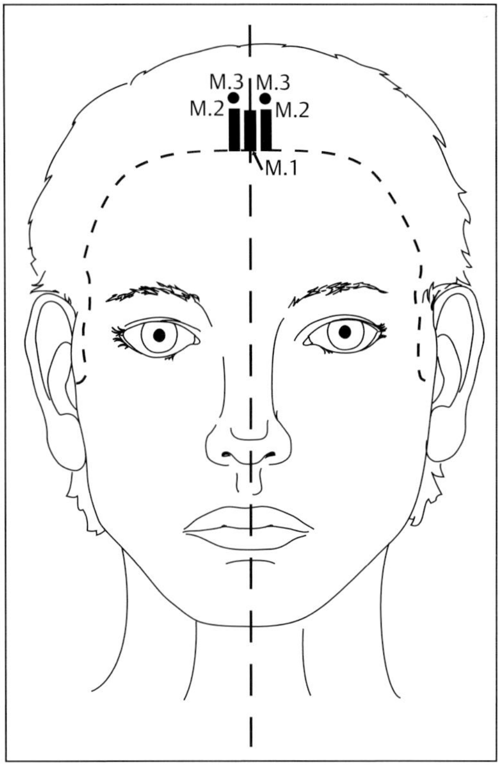

Figure 6–35 Basic points M-1–3 Yin.

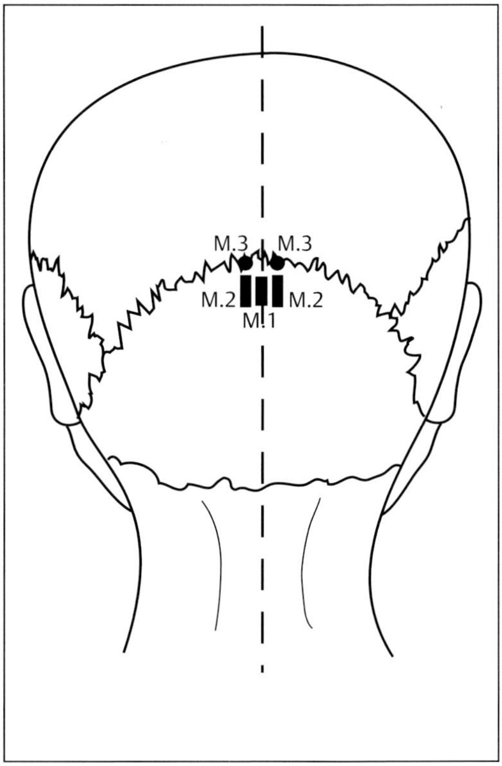

Figure 6–36 Basic points M-1–3 Yang.

Location

Yin of YIN: At the midline of the hairline over the metopic suture going 20 mm posteriorly is M-1. M-2 and M-3 are 0.25 cun lateral to the midline. M-2 is at the hairline going posteriorly 20 mm. Directly behind M-2 is M-3 going posterior another 10 mm, see **Figure 6–35**.

Yin of YANG: At the midline of the occipital over the external occipital protuberance M-1 goes anterior 15 mm. M-2 and M-3 are 0.2 cun lateral to the midline. M-2 starts along the Yin of YANG A-3, B-1, and C-1 line going anteriorly 15 mm. Directly superior-anterior to M-2 is M-3, going another 7 mm superior anteriorly; see **Figure 6–36**.

Technique

Palpate the metopic suture over the frontal bone in the midline, identify the suture ridge, and then piqué the M-1 point if needed, based on history, physical findings, and YNSA abdominal and neck diagnosis tenderness for brain point. Move laterally the prescribed fraction of a cun to palpate the little hill for M-2 and M-3. All three points may be taken individually or together, either ipsilaterally or bilaterally. The point usually is tender to palpation. Piqué subcutaneously at a 20 degree angle over the point and thread the needle over the length of the point as needed.

Purpose and Use

All upper and lower motor neuron dysfunctions, hemiplegia, paraplegia, Parkinson's disease, multiple sclerosis, hormonal dysfunction, migraine, cranial nerve entrapment neuropathies, trigeminal neuralgia, neuritis, neuropathy, vertigo, tinnitus, aphasia, visual changes, epilepsy, insomnia, dementia, depression, attention deficit disorder (ADD), Alzheimer's disease, fatigue, temporal mandibular joint (TMJ) dysfunction, and tension cephalgia.

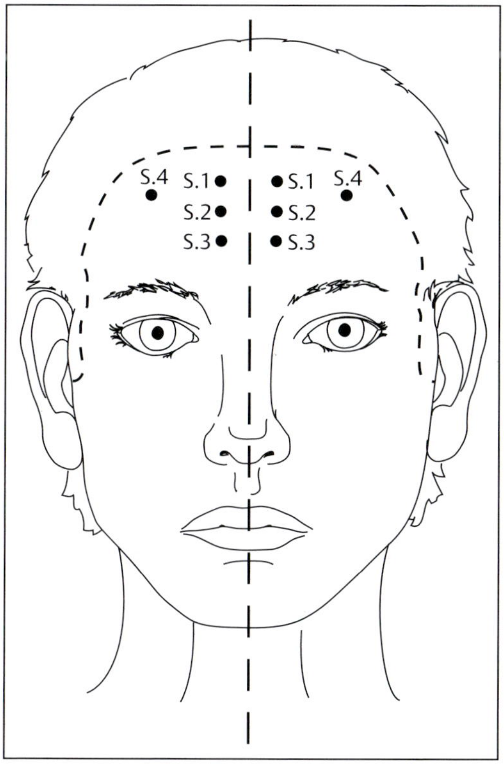

Figure 6–37 Basic points S-1–4 Yin.

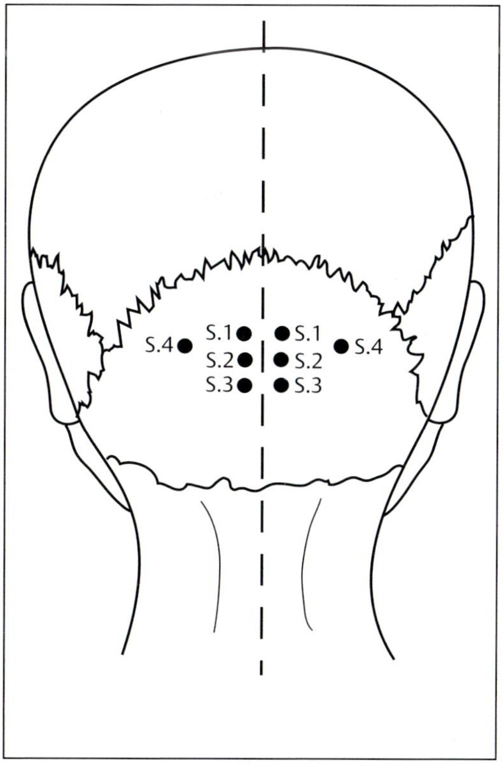

Figure 6–38 Basic points S-1–4 Yang.

Points S-1–4

Anatomical Correlate

Ipsilateral: Points S-1–4 are named for special senses. The eye is S-1, nose is S-2, mouth is S-3, and ear is S-4.

Location

Yin of YIN: S-1 is located 0.5 cun lateral to the midline and 0.5 cun below the hairline. S-2 is located 0.5 cun lateral to the midline and 1 cun below the hairline. S-3 is located 0.5 cun lateral to the midline and 1.5 cun below the hairline. S-4 is located 0.7 cun below the hairline and 0.25 cun medial to the C-1 line, see **Figure 6–37**. All these points are little hills on palpation, 2 to 3 mm in length.

Yin of YANG: On the occiput, S-1 is located ~0.3 cun lateral to the midline and 0.3 cun inferior to the Yang hairline points A-3, B-1, and C-1. Point S-2 is 0.3 lateral to the midline and 0.6 cun inferior from the Yang points A-3, B-1, C-1. S-3 is located 0.3 cun lateral to the midline and 1 cun inferior to the Yang A-3, B-1, and C-1 line. S-4 is located between the S-1 and S-2 points and medial C-1 line, see **Figure 6–38**. Points S-1–4 are ~2–3 mm in length.

Technique

Palpate the little hill; press with fingernail to illicit tenderness. Then piqué the point needed, S-1, S-2, S-3, and S-4, or all four points individually, depending on tenderness to palpation. Piqué subcutaneously at a 70 degree angle over the point(s).

Purpose and Use

- S-1 eye point: impaired vision, glaucoma, ocular pain, conjunctivitis esophoria and exophoria, strabismus sprain, strains, and somatic dysfunction, pre- and postoperative ocular pain.

- S-2 nose point: asnomia, rhinitis, sinusitis, allergic conditions, nasal obstruction, somatic dysfunction, pre- and postoperative nasal procedures.
- S-3 mouth point: aphasia, tooth and gum pain, stomatitis, herpes simplex, tonsillitis, pharyngitis, somatic dysfunction, temporal mandibular joint pain, pre- and postoperative oral pain.
- S-4 ear point: otitis media, otitis externa, tinnitus, somatic dysfunction, pre- and postoperative otic pain.

Basic Point Summary

There are 23 Basic points that appear on the front and back, left and right side of the scalp. They are further represented in the YIN, which is the anterior half of the scalp, and their corresponding/ mirror image 23 Basic points are also found in the YANG, posterior half of the scalp. Of the 23 Basic points described, five Basic points have subdivisions, which relate to individual vertebral units or parts of the appendicular system.

The Basic points are the starting point for most YNSA treatment. By identifying the body part that is diseased or dysfunctional through history and physical examination or medical investigation, a YNSA physician can then appropriately approach the patient. Basic points are primarily used to treat neuromusculoskeletal pain and dysfunction. Dramatic effects occur in newly acquired motor/sensory nerve pathology such as paraplegia, hemiplegia, sciatica, herniated disc, and, to a lesser extent, inflammatory conditions and internal organ dysfunction and disease. The four sensory points S-1–4 are used to treat all manner of illness and dysfunction of these organs: eyes, ears, nose, and mouth. The three brain points are best used to treat central nervous system disorders. The three special points for tinnitus, aphasia, and TMJ will be discussed in Chapter 8.

YNSA Somatotope of the Chest Basic Points

Dr. Toshikatsu Yamamoto discovered the YNSA somatotope on the scalp. He then went on to identify YNSA Basic points in two additional somatotopes: the chest and pubis area of the lower abdomen.

As illustrated in **Figure 6–39**, chest Basic points are identified with the brain point over the manubrium and the cervical spine just inferior to the manubrium parallel to the midline ipsilaterally. The shoulder joint is over the sternocostal junction of the first rib. The thoracic spine is over the sternocostal junction of the second and third ribs. The lumbar spine is over the sternocostal junction of the fourth rib. The thigh is in the innerspace between the fourth and fifth ribs. The knee is over the sternocostal space of the fifth rib. The lower leg is just inferior to the fifth rib. The foot is located over the sternocostal junction of the seventh rib by the zyphoid process.

YNSA Somatotope of the Pubis Basic Points

The YNSA somatotope of the pubis, see **Figure 6–40**, was identified by Dr. Toshikatsu Yamamoto, with M-1, M-2, M-3 over the pubic symphysis. The A point cervical region is just lateral to the pubic symphysis. Lateral to that point, or 0.5 cun from the pubic symphysis, is the B point for the shoulder, and 0.5 cun directly lateral to that is point C, which is ~1 cun lateral to the pubic symphysis. Points D-1–6 are 1.5 cun lateral to the pubic symphysis. Points E-1–12 are located 1 cun superior to point A and travel at a 15 degree angle ~30 mm.

The alternative somatotopes of the chest and the pubis listed here are infrequently used. When scalp positions are not readily available for various reasons, the chest or pubis YNSA Basic points would work just as well as the scalp. These alternative somatotopes are also useful when repeated use of the scalp acupoint renders that area too tender or less than 100% effective for relief of pain.

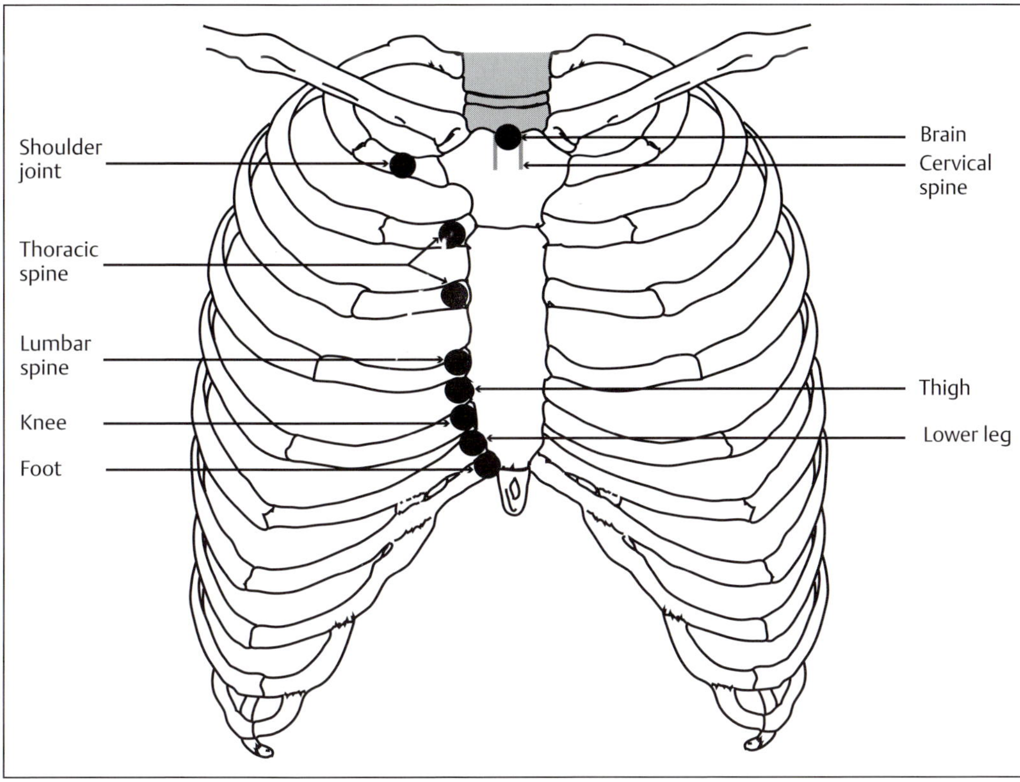

Figure 6–39 Chest somatotope.

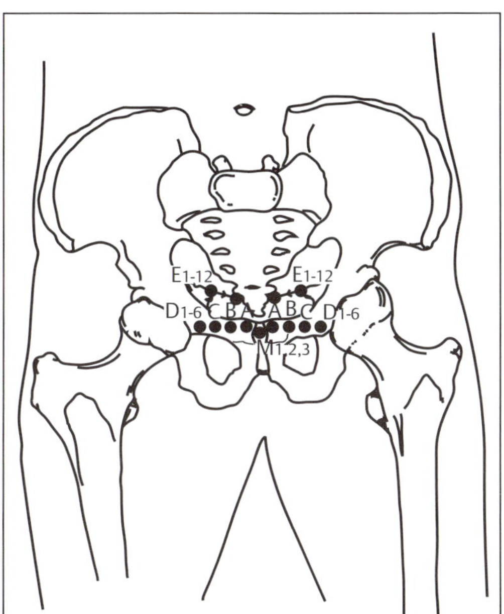

Figure 6–40 Pubis somatotope.

Summary

YNSA Basic points correspond to anatomical body parts. YNSA Basic points are found in all four quadrants directly relating to disease progression. They are Yin of YIN, Yang of YIN, Yin of YANG, and Yang of YANG. YNSA Basic points are the first points used. They may be used with any disease or condition for which YNSA is indicated.

There are Basic points identified in the chest and the pubis that may be used instead of the scalp Basic points. They may be used at the physician's preference, especially if the health problem is closer to the chest or pubis, and more importantly if the scalp points do not completely remove the pain.

震 ䷲ 震 ***Zhèn***

Taking Action—Thunder Above, Thunder Below

"Sequence of the Gua: For taking charge of a sacrificial vessel, no one is more suitable than the eldest son. Thus, after Establishing the New, Taking Action follows.
Decision
Taking Action.
Prosperous and smooth.
Thunder comes – alarm! alarm!
Laughing and talking – ha, ha!
Thunder shocks a hundred li.
The sacrificial spoon and chalice do not fall."
Thunder is dual.
Action is doubled.
In correspondence with this,
The superior person with fearful mind
Is cultivating his virtue and examining his fault.[2]

References

Acupoint schema and charts are found in on page 144 f.

1. Zheng-cai L, et al. A Study of Daoist Acupuncture and Moxibustion. Boulder, CO: Blue Poppy Press; 1999: 41
2. Huang A. The Complete I Ching. Rochester, VT: Inner Traditions; 1998: 405–407

7

YNSA Ypsilon Points – Channel Points

"It is by virtue of the twelve channels that human life exist[s,] that diseases arise, that human beings can be treated and illnesses cured. The twelve channels are where beginners start and masters end. To beginners it seems easy. The masters know how difficult it is. Qi cannot travel without a path just as water flows or the sun and moon orbit without rest so do the yin *vessels nourish the* zang *and the* yang *vessels nourish the* fu*." – Su Wen*

"Experience is a comb which nature gives to men when they are bald." – Chinese Proverb

Ypsilon points. Named after Yamamoto for the 12 channels found on the side of the head in the four left and four right quadrants.

Channels. The Chinese discovered 12 channels in which *qi* flows. YNSA can be used to treat a myriad of channel-based problems with just a few needles.

YNSA Ypsilon Points

The 12 Ypsilon points correspond to the 12 major Traditional Chinese Medicine (TCM) channels, and they relate to TCM and Five Phase diagnosis and treatment. These 12 Ypsilon points may be used whenever TCM or Five Phase channels need to be used. The 12 Ypsilon points are present in all four quadrants of the head, both left and right. These points were named and numbered by Dr. Yamamoto. YNSA neck diagnosis corresponds to the TCM and Five Phase pulse diagnosis regarding channel repletion (excess) and/or vacuity (deficiency). YNSA diagnostic and treatment methods may be used as stand-alone diagnostics and stand-alone treatment, or YNSA points may be used in conjunction with body acupuncture modalities such as TCM, Five Phase and Energetics (French) acupuncture treatments. **Table 7–1** lists the channels/YNSA point order. Yamamoto started out with the small intestine and finished with the heart. TCM states that the *qi* starts at the lung and Five Phase system numbers the channels starting with the heart, following the Chinese clock of *qi* flow. Feely numbered the channels according to the way one would identify the Ypsilon points on the side of the head, starting with the gall bladder moving up the line to the liver, then the heart and across to the pericardium, next the lung, then on the second line finding the spleen, stomach, and small intestine points, then on to the lower horizontal line identifying the kidney, bladder, triple burner, and large intestine.

Table 7–1 Channel/Ypsilon point order

Yamamoto	Feely	TCM	Five Phase
Y1 = SI	GB = Y7	LU = Y10	HT = Y12
Y2 = TB	LR = Y5	LI = Y3	SI = Y1
Y3 = LI	HT = Y12	ST = Y4	BL = Y9
Y4 = ST	PC = Y11	SP = Y6	KI = Y8
Y5 = LR	LU = Y10	HT = Y12	PC = Y11
Y6 = SP	SP = Y6	SI = Y1	TB = Y2
Y7 = GB	ST = Y4	BL = Y9	GB = Y7
Y8 = KI	SI = Y1	KI = Y8	LR = Y5
Y9 = BL	KI = Y8	PC = Y11	LU = Y10
Y10 = LU	BL = Y9	TB = Y2	LI = Y 3
Y11 = PC	TB = Y2	GB = Y7	ST = Y4
Y12 = HT	LI = Y3	LR = Y5	SP = Y6

History of Channel Theory

The history of how Channel theory was developed in TCM body acupuncture is that different theories were advanced to explain the discovery of these channels. There are two basic types of theories: points first and channels second or channels first and points second. According to the first theory, there were centuries of observation of tender points in the body—during the course of disease and as the symptoms were alleviated with the use of massage and heat. Initially the points were tabulated as their relationships were discovered, then they were linked into groups of common characteristics and effects. They then developed pathways of channels. According to the second theory—channels first and points second—the propagation of sensation during the course of massage and the exploration of internal structures through meditation and *qi gong* practice led to the discovery of the pathways or channels, with knowledge of the specific points coming later. During the excavation of the Western Han dynasty tomb Mawangdui, a silk book was discovered containing information that describes the pathways of 11 channels but does not refer to any specific points.

The functions of these channels are:

(1) transporting *qi* and blood to the body, thus rendering the body an integrated whole, (2) protecting the body, (3) responding to dysfunction in the body, and (4) transmitting *qi* to the diseased area. The complex interweaving network of channels provides transportation of *qi* and blood to every part of the body. All the sense organs and tissues are nourished, energized, and warmed by *qi* and blood.

The analogy of the plant may be helpful in understanding the channels and their organs. The *zang fu* (solid and hollow) organs may be perceived as the roots of the channels. These channels themselves are the stems, and the different body tissues with the sense organs are flowers. These channels have numerous interconnections. For example, the primary lung channel originates in the stomach and passes through the large intestine and the diaphragm, whereas the primary channel of the heart connects with the small intestine and lung. This theory of the channels underlines one of the most significant studies of Chinese medicine. The channels form the physiological interconnections that render the body an integrated whole rather than independent units, with the dense connection of channels in the scalp and head. Individual channels may be identified and stimulated to affect an entire area and organ with just one needle using YNSA methodologies.

The *Su Wen* says, "When the pathogen comes to dwell as a guest, first it resides in the skin and the body hair. If it remains and does not leave, it will enter the minute connecting channels. If it remains and does not leave, it will enter the *luo* connecting channels. If it remains and does not leave, it will enter the channels reaching the five *zang* and spreading into the intestines and into the stomach." Various kinds of channels occupy different depths within the body and act as nourishing vessels to provide energy in different layers of the body, preventing penetration of pathogens. Wind, cold, damp, heat, fire, and dryness are important causes for disease according to Traditional Chinese Medicine. When extreme, with the body's resistance low, these climatic conditions can effectively penetrate the body into the deeper levels such as the *zang fu* organs, bones, and joints. This penetration into the deep layers causes serious disease. It is from this Chinese medical philosophy that we get the four phases of disease as it travels from superficial to deep in the human body.

Drs. Paul Nogier and Toshikatsu Yamamoto have identified four phases in their respective microsystems, auricular and scalp. These four phases have been correlated with the progression of illness from superficial to intermediate to deep to spiritual essence. Dr. Nogier has identified three phases in the front of the ear and one phase on the back of the ear. Dr. Yamamoto identified Ypsilon and Basic points that have four phases. Using the Ypsilon points as an example, when an acute illness comes on, the treatment frequently is Yin of YIN. Then, as it progresses deeper into the body, the phase changes to Yang of YIN, then to Yin of YANG, and finally, to Yang of YANG—when here, it has progressed deeply into the person to affect spirit and psyche of the individual. As the illness penetrates deeper into the body, the YNSA treatment approach requires needle placement at the properly selected phase or quadrant.

Relationship of Channels and Body Dysfunction

TCM and YNSA promote harmony and balance within the energetic body system. When the harmony of the body is disrupted due to any cause or disease, the channel can respond in any number of ways. First, when there is disease in the channels themselves, you have local tenderness, pain, weakness, distention, numbness, and tingling. This disease of the membrane means there is impaired flow of *qi* or blood, which is stagnation or insufficiency of *qi* and blood leading to malnourishment at the cellular level and progressing up to the organ level. Second, when the *zang fu* organs have become injured, depending on the kind of injury, the disorder can then relate anywhere along the acupuncture channel. Diseases can then be transmitted via the channels, passing from one *zang fu* organ to another. Finally, in some cases, in the course of the disease the channel can be discolored and visible, showing a purple color indicating heat due to stasis of blood, or a pale color as a result of a vacuity of *qi* and blood.

The acupuncture channels serve as conduits to transmit acupuncture's stimulation of *qi* from the acupuncture point to the diseased area of the body, rendering the acupuncture treatment effective. This is done by the needle stimulating body acupuncture points electrically, then biochemically, thereby regulating the flow of *qi* and blood in the whole course of the channel.[1] The same can be said of microsystem treatments and of YNSA in particular.

The Twelve Primary Acupuncture Channels

The 12 primary channels run vertically bilaterally and symmetrically. Each channel corresponds to and connects internally with one of the *zang fu* organs as shown in **Table 2–2** in Chapter 2. These channels correspond to the *zang* organs that are *yin* and the *fu* organs that are *yang*. There are six *yin* organs and five *yang* organs. Triple burner (TB) is a *yang* channel without a physical organ, so there are six *yin* and six *yang* channels. There are three *yin* channels and three *yang* channels in the arm. There are three *yin* channels and three *yang* channels in the leg. The *yang* channels traverse the outer surface of the arm or the leg and travel to the head.

The *yin* channels traverse the inner surface of the limbs, abdomen, and chest. The three *yin* channels of the hand: lung (LU), pericardium (PC), or heart (HT) begin in the chest and travel along the inner surface of the arm to the hand. Three *yang* channels of the hand are large intestine (LI), triple burner (TB), and small intestine (SI). They begin in the hand and travel along the outer surface of the arm to the head.

The three *yang* channels of the foot are the stomach (ST), gall bladder (GB), and bladder (BL). They begin on the face in the region of the eye and travel down along the body on the outer surface of the leg to the foot. The three *yin* channels of the foot are the spleen (SP), liver (LR), and kidney (KI). They begin in the foot and travel along the inner surface of the leg or the flank. These 12 channels comprise the internal and external pathways of *qi* and blood. The external pathway is what is normally shown on most acupuncture charts and is superficial. All the acupuncture points of the channel lie on the external pathway. The internal pathways are the deep paths of the channels that enter the body cavities and are not accessible for acupuncture needling.

The naming of each of the 12 channels is based on the *zang* (solid) or *fu* (hollow) organs to which it belongs, second, the limb, upper or lower, through which it traverses, and its *yin* or *yang* identity.

There are 12 divergent channels that branch out from the primary channels and have no specific points of their own. Pathways make internal linkages that may not be made by the primary channels. Divergent channels belong to the *yang* primary channels, the interrelated *zang* or *fu* organs, as well as their internally or externally related channels. The divergent channels strengthen the *yin* and *yang* relationship between the internally and externally related channels in *zang fu*. They also distribute *qi* and blood to the head and face. They integrate parts of the body that are not supplied or connected to the primary channels.

Eight Extraordinary Vessels

Besides the 12 primary channels and 12 divergent channels, there are eight extraordinary vessels or curious channels. These extraordinary vessels are conception (*ren mai*), the governing (*du mai*), the penetrating (*chong mai*), the girdle (*dai mai*), the *yin* motility (*yin qiao*), and the *yang* motility (*yang qiao*), the yin linking (*yin wei*), and the yang linking (*yang wei*). Of the eight extraordinary vessels, only the conception and governing vessels have their own acupuncture points. The others use points of the 12 primary channels.

The extraordinary vessels act as reservoirs to absorb repletion *qi* and blood from the primary channels. The extraordinary vessels link the 12 primary channels, forming various pools or seas, the sea of yang channels, the sea of *yin* channels, the sea of blood, the sea of *qi*, the sea of marrow, and the sea of nourishment. The girdle vessel (*dai mai*) encircles the body at the waist, binding the vertical paths of the 12 primary channels. The *yin* motility (*yin qiao*) is said to dominate quietness in the body. The *yang* motility (*yang qiao*) is said to dominate activity of the body. The *yin* linking (*yin wei*) is said to dominate the interior parts of the body. The *yang* linking (*yang wei*) is said to dominate the exterior parts of the body.

The extraordinary vessels protect the body as a defensive *qi* for the chest, abdomen, and back from any exterior pathological factors. It is these three extraordinary vessels, conception (*ren mai*), governing (*du mai*), and penetrating (*chong mai*), that originate in the pelvic cavity and are directly linked to the kidneys, which are the storehouse of preheaven *qi*. This function of the extraordinary vessels brings to light the relationship between the constitutional vigor and the defense against disease. There are other channels that do not particularly relate directly to YNSA at this point, such as *luo* connecting channels. The rest of the point categories of TCM are not directly related to YNSA and will not be discussed.

Twelve Primary Channel Pathways and Pathology

This section is designed for the practitioner who is not completely familiar with TCM or how the TCM practitioner thinks about the acupuncture channel and the related organ. By learning these characteristics, one would easily further investigate the possibility of using YNSA neck diagnosis or abdominal diagnosis to confirm the necessity of treating the Ypsilon point relating to these 12 channels, thus using one needle to treat the whole. By studying these pathological signs and symptoms, one is able to then predict the probability of finding a positive YNSA neck diagnosis and tender Ypsilon point. Andrew Ellis, Nigel Wiseman, and Ken Boss in their book, *Fundamentals of Chinese Acupuncture*, provide a wonderful description of the flow of *qi* through the channels, and their description is greatly relied upon in the following discussions.[2]

Lung Channel—Hand *Tai Yin*

This primary lung channel starts in the region of the stomach in the middle burner (*jiao*) and descends to connect to the large intestine. It returns upward passing the opening of the stomach and penetrating the diaphragm, and goes to the lung, its home. The lung channel continues to ascend the respiratory tract into the throat and moves laterally toward the clavicle into the axilla. From here it runs down the anterior aspect of the upper arm, lateral to the heart and pericardium channels. It traverses the cubital fossa and continues along the anterior aspect of the forearm to the radial styloid process at the wrist. It crosses the radial pulse, traverses the thenar eminence, and travels along the radial side of the thumb to its tip at the nail.

Main Pathological Signs Associated with the External Path of the Lung Channel

Fever and an aversion to cold with or without sweating. There is nasal congestion, headache, pain in the supraclavicular fossa, pain in the shoulders, chest, and back, cold pain along the channel of the arm.

Main Pathological Signs Associated with the Internal Path of the Lung Channel

Coughing, wheezing, dyspnea, rapid breathing, fullness of the chest and oppression in the chest, expectoration of phlegm, dry throat, abnormal urine color, restlessness, coughing up of blood, heat in the palms of the hands.

Distal Effects

Distention of the abdomen and thin stool or diarrhea. Repletion of lung *qi* is associated with back pain, wind-cold contraction with spontaneous sweating, frequent urination, and yawning. Insufficiency of lung *qi* is associated with shoulder and back pain accompanied by fear of cold, shortness of breath, distressed rapid breathing, and abnormal color of the urine.

Large Intestine Channel—Hand *Yang Ming*

The primary large intestine channel pathway. The hand *yang ming* large intestine channel begins at the radial side of the tip of the index finger and proceeds upward between the first and second metacarpal bones of the hand. It then traverses between the tendons of the extensor pollicis longus and brevis at the wrist. It continues along the radial margin of the forearm to the lateral aspect of the elbow and then up the lateral aspect of the upper arm over the shoulder. After intersection with the hand *tai yang* small intestine channel at SI-12, it rises to just below the spinous process of the seventh cervical vertebra and intersects the governing vessel at GV-14. GV-14 is where all six *yang* channels meet. The large intestine channel then travels straight to the supraclavicular fossa and ST-12; from there it connects through the lung and passes through the diaphragm and goes directly to the large intestine, its home.

Main Pathological Signs Associated with the External Path of the Large Intestine Channel

Fever, parched dry mouth, and thirst, sore throat, nose bleed, tooth ache, pain or redness of the eyes, swelling of the neck, palpable red swelling and inhibited movement of the fingers. There is pain and sensation of cold or painful, palpably hot, red, swollen shoulder and upper arm.

Main Pathological Signs Associated with the Internal Path of the Large Intestine Channel

Abdominal pain; migrating abdominal pain; thin stool; slimy, sticky, yellow stool; rapid breathing; and dyspnea. Repletion of large intestine *qi* causes distention, swelling, and heat along the course of the channel. Insufficiency of large intestine *qi* causes cold and shivering with an inability to regain warmth.

Distal Effects

Spasm, stiffness, and pain or strain along the course of the large intestine channel with the inability to raise the arm or rotate the neck left or right.

Stomach Channel—Foot *Yang Ming*

The primary stomach channel. The foot *yang ming* stomach channel starts at the side of the nose then ascends to the inner canthus of the eye to intersect with the foot *tai yang* bladder channel at BL-1. It then descends parallel to the nose, penetrates the axilla into the upper gum, and joins the governing vessel at GV-26. It skirts back along the upper and lower lips to join the conception vessel at CV-24 in the mentolabial groove of the chin. It then runs along the mandible to ST-5 and rounds the angle of the mandible to ST-6. It proceeds upward in front of the ear and intersects the foot *shao yang* gall bladder channel at GB-3 and continues along the hairline. It then intersects the foot *shao yang* channel again at GB-6 and crosses the midline of the forehead and intersects with the governing vessel at GV-24.

Main Pathological Signs Associated with the External Path of the Stomach Channel

High fever, flushed face, sweating, clouding of the spirit, delirium, manic agitation, aversion to cold, pain in the eyes, dry nose, nose bleed, lesion of the lips and in the mouth, sore larynx swollen at the neck, stiff neck, chest pain, cold or pain, redness or swelling of the lower limbs.

Main Pathological Signs Associated with the Internal Path of the Stomach Channel

Pronounced abdominal distention, fullness and edema, restlessness and discomfort while active or recumbent, mania or withdrawal. There can also be rapid hunger, yellow urine, and hypersecretion of the stomach. Repletion stomach *qi* gives rise to heat in the anterior aspect of the body, persistent hunger, and yellow urine. Insufficient stomach *qi* produces cold in the anterior aspect of the body, shivering, and stomach cold resulting in distention and fullness. The main musculoskeletal pathological signs include strained middle toe, spasms in the lower leg, hardened muscles in the foot, pain and spasms in the thigh muscles, pain and swelling in the inguinal area, abdominal tension and spasm extending to the neck and the jaw, dryness of the mouth, spasm with inability to close the eye, heat with inability to open the eye, abnormal stimulation of the orbicularis oris muscle causing abnormal mouth position.

Spleen Channel—Foot *Tai Yin*

The primary spleen channel. The foot *tai yin* spleen channel starts on the medial tip of the great toe and runs along the border of the light and dark skin of the medial aspect of the foot. It traverses in front of the medial malleolus and up the posterior side of the leg along the posterior margin of the tibia. The spleen channel then runs anterior to the foot *jue yin* liver channel passing medial to the knee and up the anterior medial abdomen and intersects the conception vessel at CV-3 and CV-4 before going to the spleen, its home, and connecting with the stomach. This channel then continues upward and passes through the diaphragm to intersect with the foot *shao yang* gall bladder at GB-24 and the foot *jue yin* liver at LR-14. From there it descends to the side of the esophagus and crosses the hand *tai yin* lung channel at LU-1 and finally proceeds up to the root of the tongue to disperse over its lower surface.

Main Pathological Signs Associated with the External Path of the Spleen Channel

Heaviness in the head and body, fatigue and weakness of the limbs, general fever, pain in the posterior mandibular region of the lower cheek, motor impairment of the tongue, wasting and atrophy of the muscles and limbs, cold along the inside of the thigh and knee, edema, swelling of the legs and feet.

Main Pathological Signs Associated with the Internal Path of the Spleen Channel

Pain in the ventral area of the abdomen, thin diarrhea or stool containing undigested food, nausea and vomiting, lower abdominal lump, reduced food intake, jaundice, inhibited urination. Signs of repletion spleen *qi* are spasms and foot pain. Signs of insufficiency of spleen *qi* cause abdominal fullness, intestinal rumbling, undigested food, and diarrhea.

Distal Effects

Strain of the large toe, pain in the medial malleolus, pain or cramp in the gastrocnemius, pain in the medial aspect of the knee, pain in the inner thigh and inguinal region, cutting pain in the genitals.

Heart Channel—Hand *Shao Yin*

The primary heart channel. The hand *shao yin* heart channel starts in the heart, merging with the blood vessels surrounding the organ; traveling downward it passes through the diaphragm to connect to the small intestine.

Main Pathological Signs Associated with the External Path of the Heart Channel

General fever, headache, pain in the eyes, chest, back muscles, dry throat with the urge to drink, hot or painful palms of the hands and feet, pain in the scapular region and/or the medial aspect of the forearm.

Main Pathological Signs Associated with the Internal Path of the Heart Channel

Cardiac chest pain, fullness and pain in the chest and lateral costal region, pain in the hypochondriac region, rapid breathing, discomfort when recumbent, dizziness with fainting, essence-spirit disorders.

Distal Effects

Internal tension or cramping, infracardiac deep pain, pain and cramping as a strain along the inner aspect of the medial arm.

Small Intestine Channel—Hand *Tai Yin*

The primary small intestine channel. The hand *tai yin* small intestine channel starts in the outside edge of the little finger tip and travels along the ulnar side of the hand to the wrist, merging in the ulnar styloid process. It then continues up the posterior aspect of the metacarpal lunate bone. It passes between the olecranon to the ulnar and the medial epicondyle of the humerus on the medial side of the elbow. The small intestine channel then runs up the posterior medial side of the upper arm, emerging behind the shoulder and circling around the inferior fossa to the superior fossa of the scapula. At the top of shoulder it intersects with the foot *tai yang* bladder channel at BL-41 and BL-11, connecting with the governing vessel at GV-14 before turning downward to the supraclavicular fossa. Here it submerges and connects with the heart and follows with the esophagus down through the diaphragm to the stomach. It then intersects with the conception vessel internally at CV-13 and CV-12 before going to the small intestine itself, its home.

Main Pathological Signs Associated with the External Path of the Small Intestine

Erosion of the glossal and oral mucosa, pain in the cheeks, sore pharynx, lachrymation, stiffness of the neck, pain in the lateral aspect of the shoulders and upper arm.

Main Pathological Signs Associated with the Internal Path of the Small Intestine

Lower abdominal pain and distention, pain stretching around the lumbar region, lower abdominal pain radiating into the testicles, diarrhea, pain in the stomach with dry feces and constipation.

Distal Effects

Strain and inability to support the little finger, pain in the lateral aspect of the elbow, pain in the medial aspect of the upper arm and axilla, axilla pain that extends back over the scapula and neck, tinnitus, pain in the ear, pain in the submandibular region, the need to close the eyes for a while before one can get them to focus, spasm and tension in the neck resulting in swelling.

Bladder Channel—Foot *Tai Yang*

The primary urinary bladder channel is as follows: the foot *tai yang* bladder channel starts in the inner canthus of the eye and travels upward over the forehead intersecting the governing vessel at GV-24 and the foot *shao yang* gall bladder channel at GB-25 and GB-15. It travels up to the vertex of the head and again meets with the governing vessel at GV-20. From the vertex, a branch descends from the temple and the region around the ear intersecting GB-7, GB-8, GB-9, GB-10, GB-11, and GB-12. From the vertex, another branch enters the brain, meets DU-17, and emerges to descend to the nape of the neck where the channel splits into two branches. The medial branch descends along the posterior aspect of the neck, intersecting with DU-14 and DU-13. It descends along the spine 1.5 cun lateral to the midline all the way down to the lumbar region. It penetrates deep into the paravertebral muscles connecting with the kidneys and linking with the bladder. It further descends from the lumbar region into the sacrum, crosses the buttocks, and descends to the popliteal fossa of the knee at BL-40. The lateral branch descends from the nape of the neck to the medial border of the scapula and then parallel to the spine 3 cun lateral to the midline all the way to the gluteal region. It then crosses the buttocks, intersects with GB-30, then descends along the posterior aspect of the thigh meeting up at the popliteal fossa and BL-40. It travels down the gastrocnemius muscle and emerges at BL-60 at the lateral malleolus along the fifth metatarsal bone ending at BL-67 on the lateral side of the tip of the fifth toe.

Main Pathological Signs Associated with the External Path of the Bladder Channel

Chills and fever; headache; stiff neck; pain in the cervical, thoracic, and lumbar regions along the spine; ocular pain and lachrymation; and pain in the posterior thigh, popliteal region, gastrocnemius, and foot.

Main Pathological Signs Associated with the Internal Path of the Bladder Channel

Pain and distention in the lower abdomen, inhibited micturition, urinary block and enuresis, mental disorders.

Distal Effects

Strain or inability to support the little toe, pain and swelling of the heel, spasm and tension of the popliteal region, spasm or tension in the neck, inability to raise the arm, muscular discomfort in the axilla, strained muscles in the supraclavicular fossa.

Kidney Channel—Foot *Shao Yin*

The primary kidney channel is as follows: the foot *shao yin* kidney channel starts on the underside of the little toe, crosses the sole of the foot obliquely, and emerges out of the arch of the foot under the navicular tuberosity at KI-2. It then proceeds posterior to the medial malleolus and continues into the heel. From there it travels up the rear medial aspect of the lower leg to intersect with the foot *tai yin* spleen channel at SP-6. Traveling up through the gastrocnemius muscle it ascends across the medial aspect of the popliteal fossa and the posteromedial where it meets the governing vessel at GV-1. It continues up to the link with the spinal column, up the spinal column to the kidney, its home. Afterward, it turns downward to connect with the bladder and intersect with the conception vessel at CV-4 and CV-3.

Main Pathological Signs Associated with the External Path of the Kidney Channel

Low back pain, frigidity of the legs, atrophy of the legs, dry mouth, sore pharynx, pain in the lateral gluteal region and in the posterior aspect of the thigh. There may also be pain in the soles of the feet.

Main Pathological Signs Associated with the Internal Path of the Kidney Channel

Dizziness, facial edema, ashen complexion, shortness of breath, short rapid breathing, somnolence or restlessness, enduring diarrhea, thin stool or dry stool evacuated with difficulty, nausea and vomiting, distention, and impotence.

Distal Effects

Cramping at the bottom of the foot, spasms, twisting or pain along the course of the tendons and ligaments. The major symptoms associated with these are convulsions and spasms that occur in epileptic diseases. If the disease attacks the back side of the patient, then the patient cannot bend forward. If the disease attacks the chest and abdomen side of the patient, then the patient cannot lean forward. In the *yang* diseases, the upper body curves backward. In the *yin* diseases, the upper body curves forward.

Pericardium Channel—Hand *Jue Yin*

The primary pericardium channel is as follows: the hand *jue yin* pericardium channel starts in the chest where its home is. Descending through the diaphragm into the abdomen, it connects successively to the upper, middle, and lower burners. It then runs horizontally from the center of the chest to the axilla, down the medial aspect of the upper arm into the forearm between the tendons of the pulmarus longus muscle and the flexor carpi radialis muscle. It traverses through the palm to the tip of the middle finger.

Main Pathological Signs Associated with the External Path of the Pericardium Channel

Stiffness in the neck, spasm in the limbs, red facial complexion, pain in the eyes, subaxillary swelling, hypertonicity of the elbow and arm-inhibiting movement, and hot palms of the hands.

Main Pathological Signs Associated with the Internal Path of the Pericardium Channel

Delirious speech, clouding inversion, vexation, fullness and oppression in the chest and lateral costal region, aphasia, palpitations, heart pain, constant laughter, and other essence-spirit disorders.

Triple Burner Channel—Hand *Shao Yang*

The primary triple burner channel is as follows: the hand *shao yang* triple burner channel starts in the ulnar side of the tip of the fourth finger and travels up between the fourth and fifth metacarpal bones on the dorsum of the hand to the outside of the wrist. It then proceeds up the posterior midline of the forearm between the radius and the ulna. It runs over the olecranon process of the elbow and then travels up the posterior midline of the upper arm to the shoulder. It meets the hand *tai yang* small intestine channel at SI-12 and then runs over the back to meet the governing vessel at GV-14. It crosses back over the shoulder and intersects with the foot *shao yang* gall bladder channel at GB-21 before running into the supraclavicular fossa penetrating into the interior and traveling into the midchest region to meet the conception vessel at CV-17 where it links with the pericardium. It then descends internally to its home in each of the three burners successively.

Main Pathological Signs Associated with the External Path of the Triple Burner Channel

Sore throat, pain in the cheeks, reddening of the eyes, deafness, pain behind the ears and the posterior aspect of the shoulder and the upper arm.

Main Pathological Signs Associated with the Internal Path of the Triple Burner Channel

Abdominal distention and fullness or hardness and fullness in the lower abdomen, urinary frequency and distress, edema of the skin, enuresis.

Gall Bladder Channel—Foot *Shao Yang*

The primary gall bladder channel is as follows: the foot *shao yang* gall bladder channel starts in the outer canthus of the eye and traverses the temple to TB-22. It then rises to the corner of the forehead where it intersects with the foot *yang ming* stomach channel at ST-8. Descending behind the ear it passes down the neck in front of the hand *shao yang* triple burner channel and meets the hand *tai yang* small intestine channel at SI-17. After reaching the shoulder, it turns back and runs back behind the triple burner channel to intersect the governing vessel at GV-14. It then moves parallel to the shoulder line outward to intersect with the hand *tai yang* small intestine channel at SI-12 before crossing over to ST-12 in the supraclavicular fossa.

Main Pathological Signs Associated with the External Path of the Gall Bladder Channel

Alternating fever and chills, headache, ashen complexion, ocular pain, pain under the chin, subaxillary swelling, deafness, pain in the lateral knee and tibia.

Main Pathological Signs Associated with the Internal Path of the Gall Bladder Channel

Pain in the lateral costal area, vomiting, bitter taste in the mouth, pain in the chest.

Distal Effects

Inability to support the fourth toe, strains and sprains in the outer aspect of the knee, inability to extend and bend the knee at the popliteal fossa, strains in the pelvic region in the front or the sacral coccygeal region, pain extending up to the lateral costal region or the area just below the lateral costal region, pain in the supraclavicular fossa, the side of the chest, and/or neck, inability to hold the ipsilateral eye open when turning the head, all muscle and tendon problems, from inflammation to dislocation, including sprain and strain.

Liver Channel—Foot *Jue Yin*

The primary liver channel is as follows: the primary liver foot *jue yin* channel starts on the dorsum of the great toe and runs up the foot between the first and second metatarsal bones to a point 1 cun in front of the medial malleolus. It then proceeds upward to SP-6 where it intersects with the foot *tai yin* spleen channel and the foot *shao yin* kidney channel, continuing up the medial *tai yin* spleen channel 8 cun above the medial malleolus. It then runs posterior to the channel over the knee and thigh. It connects to the foot *tai yin* spleen channel at SP-12 and SP-13, then skirts along the genitalia and penetrates the lower abdomen where it meets the conception vessel at CV-2, CV-3, and CV-4. It then ascends, moving toward the lateral aspect of the trunk to its home in the liver, and continues, to connect with the gall bladder. Continuing its upward course through the diaphragm, it disperses over the costal region and then runs up to the neck posterior to the pharynx. Entering the nasal pharynx it meets the tissues surrounding the eyes. The channel finally runs up the forehead to meet the governing vessel at the vertex of the head.

Main Pathological Signs Associated with the External Path of the Liver Channel

Headache, dizziness, blurred vision, tinnitus, fever, spasms of the limb.

Main Pathological Signs Associated with the Internal Path of the Liver Channel

Fullness and distention and pain in the costal region with lump, fullness, and thoracic oppression in the ventral part of the abdomen, abdominal pain, vomiting, jaundice, lower abdominal pain, enuresis, urinary blockage, dark yellow urine.

Distal Effects

Inability to support the great toe, pain lateral to the medial malleolus, pain in the medial aspect of the knee, pain or spasm in the medial aspect of the thigh, dysfunction of the genitalia, impotence, retraction of the genitals due to cold injury, frequent erection due to heat damage.

YNSA Ypsilon Points and the Twelve Primary Channels

The 12 Ypsilon points in their energetic representative state correlate directly to the 12 TCM channels, or TCM and Five Phase radial pulse diagnosis.[3] Ypsilon points may be used alone or with YNSA Basic points and/or with other body acupuncture approaches such as TCM, Five Phase, and Energetics (French).

YNSA Ypsilon Point Treatment

The treatment routine is to typically treat the Basic points first. If pain or other symptoms persist, then identify the need for Ypsilon points through neck diagnosis and/or pulse and/or abdominal diagnosis, see **Figures 5–1, 5–3, 5–8,** and **Table 5–1** in Chapter 5.

The decision for use of Ypsilon point YNSA treatment is based on history and physical examination, but it becomes necessary when a positive YNSA neck diagnosis is made for an Ypsilon point.

The Ypsilon points are a dense collection of acupoints found bilaterally on the lateral sides of the scalp. They occur in front of the pinna of the ear, YIN, and behind the pinna of the ear, YANG. YIN is further divided in half; the lower half of the area in front of the pinna of the ear is called Yin of YIN. The upper half in front of the pinna of the ear is called Yang of YIN. Most of the time one will be treating patients in Yin of YIN. The lateral scalp behind the pinna of the ear is called YANG. YANG is also divided in half with the upper half called Yang of YANG and the lower half called Yin of YANG, as depicted in **Figures 1–5 to 1–9** in Chapter 1.

In the author's study of low back pain of various causes, the occurrences of Ypsilon points requiring treatment per quadrant were:[4]

- Yin of YIN 86.4%; Yang of YIN 3.8%
- Yang of YANG 1.6%; Yin of YANG 8.2%

All 12 Ypsilon points occur in each quadrant. All Ypsilon points are palpable as little hills or subcutaneous thickenings of the scalp.

Ypsilon points are 12 acupoints that correlate directly with the 12 Chinese acupuncture body channels and are labeled as such in this text.

Jue yin: LR, PC; liver, pericardium

Shao yin: HT, KI; heart, kidney

Tai yin: LU, SP; lung, spleen

Shao yang: TB, GB; triple burner, gall bladder

Yang ming: LI, ST; large intestine, stomach

Tai yang: SI, BL; small intestine, urinary bladder

For the sake of clarity, the international symbols for channels will be used throughout the book for Ypsilon point identification. Toshikatsu Yamamoto uses a numbering system he developed. Four ways of thinking about the Ypsilon points are presented in **Table 7–1**. The far left column correlates the Yamamoto numbers and channel symbols. The second is the author's ordering system based upon the orderly method one palpates for the Ypsilon points on the scalp in an orderly manner to easily find each point correlated to the Yamamoto numbering system. The third is the TCM channel sequence correlated to the Yamamoto numbering system. The far right column is the Five Phase flow of *qi* correlated to the Yamamoto numbering system.

YNSA Ypsilon Point Locations

Gall Bladder (GB)

Yin of YIN Location: Found where the pinna attaches to the scalp at the superior portion and just at the hairline where the pinna attaches to the scalp, see **Figure 7–1**.

Method of Location: With the patient seated and the physician standing in front and lateral to the patient, place the left thumb over the scalp superior to the pinna of the ear, palpating for a small hill where the hairline is located and the pinna attaches.

Liver (LR)

Yin of YIN Location: Immediately superior to the gall bladder (GB) point, see **Figure 7–2**.

Method of Location: With the patient seated and the physician standing in front and lateral to the patient, place the left thumb over the gall bladder (GB), slide superior less than 0.5 cun to palpate a small hill.

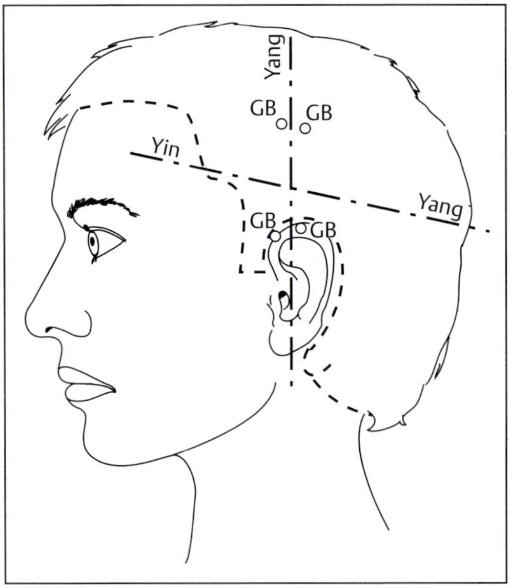

Figure 7–1 Ypsilon GB point.

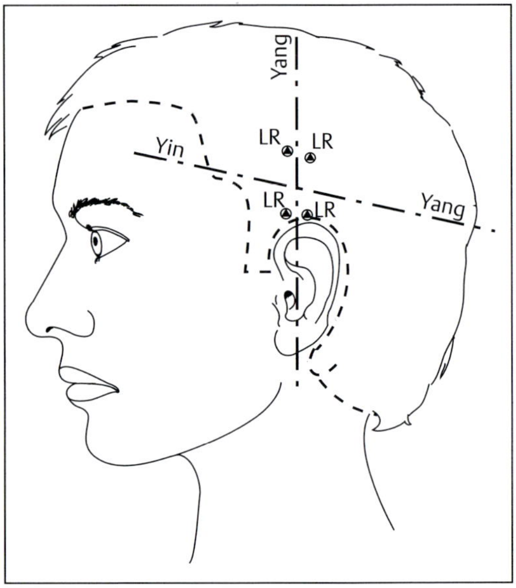

Figure 7–2 Ypsilon LR point.

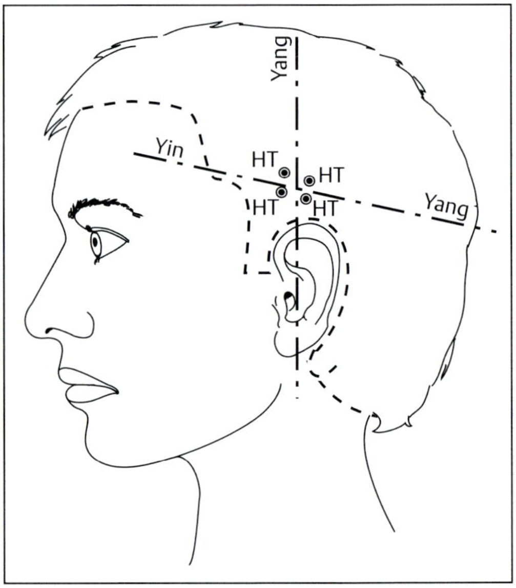

Figure 7–3 Ypsilon HT point.

Heart (HT)

Yin of YIN Location: Immediately superior to the liver (LR), see **Figure 7–3**.

Method of Location: With the patient seated and the physician standing in front and lateral to the patient, palpate the gall bladder (GB), slide up to the liver (LR), and 0.5 cun superior to the liver (LR) until a small hill is found.

Pericardium (PC)

Yin of YIN Location: 0.75 cun anterior to the heart (HT) point, see **Figure 7–4**.

Method of Location: With the patient seated and the physician standing in front and lateral to the patient, palpate the heart (HT), slide your thumb anteriorly along an ascending line of 15 degrees toward the forehead. Palpate for a small hill.

Lung (LU)

Yin of YIN Location: At the anterior hairline where it takes a posterior turn at the level of the HT and PC lines, see **Figure 7–5**.

Method of Location: With the patient seated and the physician standing in front and lateral to the patient, palpate the pericardium (PC) starting from the heart (HT), move along a line parallel to that with a 15 degree inclination anteriorly toward the hairline where the hairline changes direction. Palpate for a small hill.

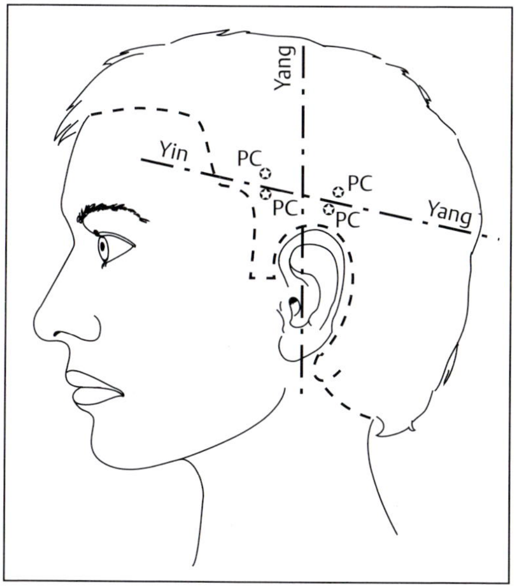

Figure 7–4 Ypsilon PC point.

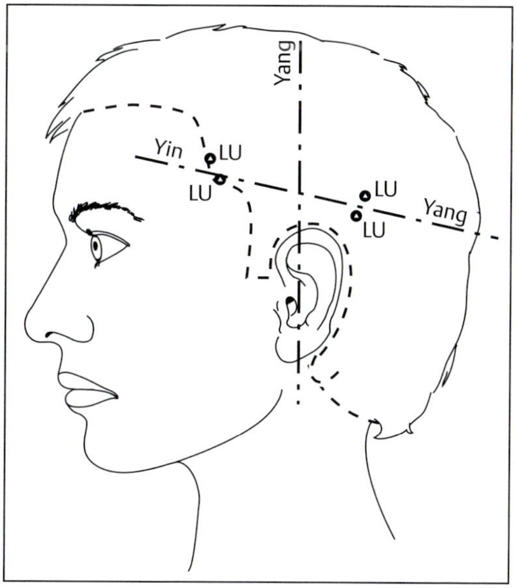

Figure 7–5 Ypsilon LU point.

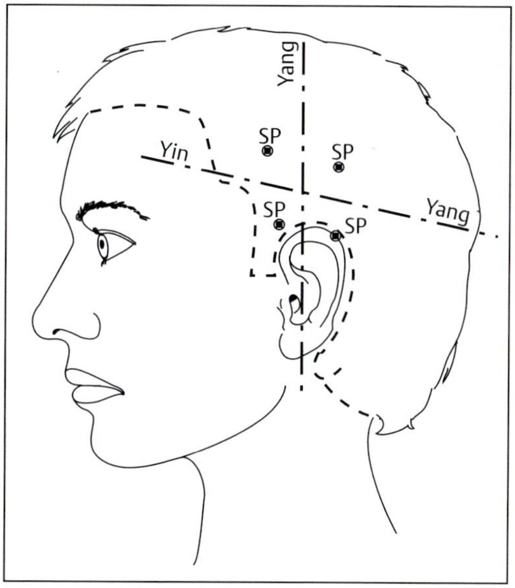

Figure 7–6 Ypsilon SP point.

Spleen (SP)

Yin of YIN Location: Anterior and inferior to the liver (LR), see **Figure 7–6**.

Method of Location: With the patient seated and the physician standing in front and lateral to the patient, palpate the gall bladder (GB), slide up to the liver (LR), and move horizontal and anterior 0.5 cun, then move palpatory finger 0.25 cun inferior to locate the small hill.

Stomach (ST)

Yin of YIN Location: Anterior to the liver (LR) and spleen (SP), see **Figure 7–7**.

Method of Location: With the patient seated and the physician standing in front and lateral to the patient, palpate the liver (LR), slide your thumb horizontally and anteriorly ~0.75 cun, and palpate a small hill.

Small Intestine (SI)

Yin of YIN Location: At the hairline, parallel to the stomach (ST), see **Figure 7–8**.

Method of Location: With the patient seated and the physician standing in front and lateral to the patient, start palpating at the gall bladder (GB), move to the liver (LR), then to the stomach (ST), and, finally, slide to the hairline in same horizontal position as the stomach (ST) to palpate a small hill.

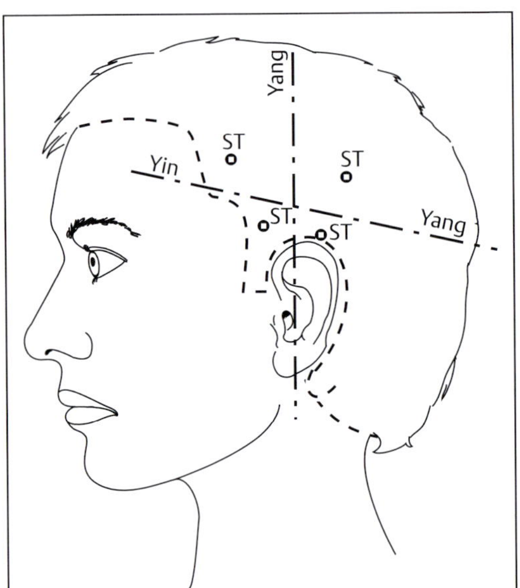

Figure 7–7 Ypsilon ST point.

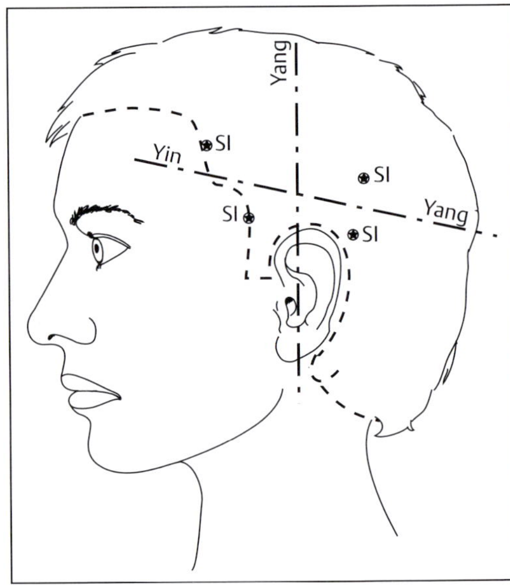

Figure 7–8 Ypsilon SI point.

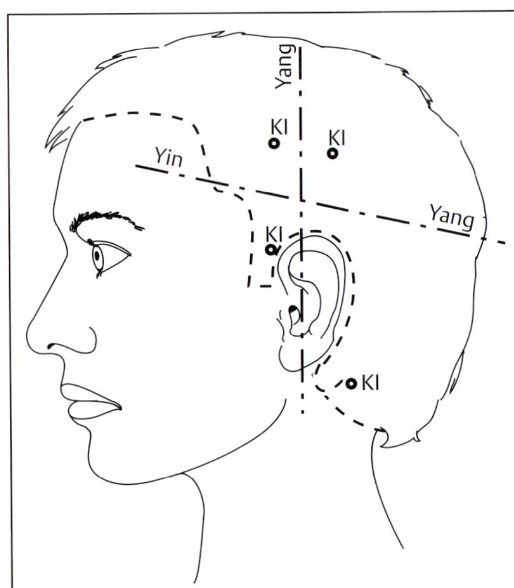

Figure 7–9 Ypsilon KI point.

Kidney (KI)

Yin of YIN Location: Anterior and inferior to the gall bladder (GB), see **Figure 7–9**.

Method of Location: With the patient seated and the physician standing in front and lateral to the patient, palpate the gall bladder (GB), slide thumb anterior 0.25 cun and inferior 0.12 cun to a small hill.

Bladder (BL)

Yin of YIN Location: Above the zygomatic process, see **Figure 7–10**.

Method of Location: With the patient seated and the physician standing in front and lateral to the patient, palpate the zygomatic process in the middle of the sideburn. There, palpate a small hill above the zygomatic process of the temporal bone in the middle of the sideburn.

Triple Burner (TB)

Yin of YIN Location: At the hairline, approximately at the height of the kidney (KI) point, see **Figure 7–11**.

Method of Location: With the patient seated and the physician standing in front and lateral to the patient, palpate the zygomatic process at the anterior sideburn hairline, slide your thumb up 0.25 cun to palpate a small hill.

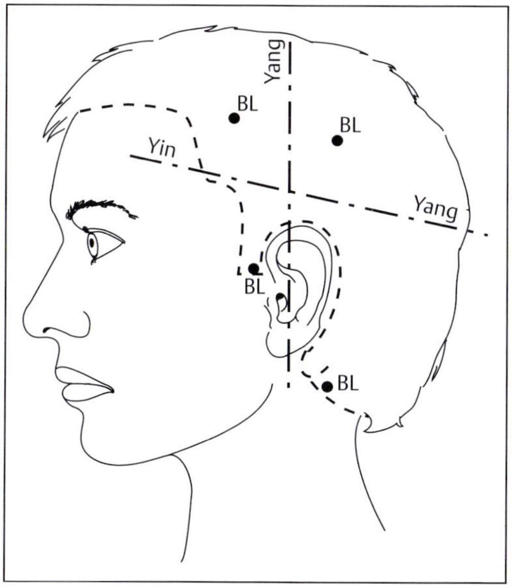

Figure 7–10 Ypsilon BL point.

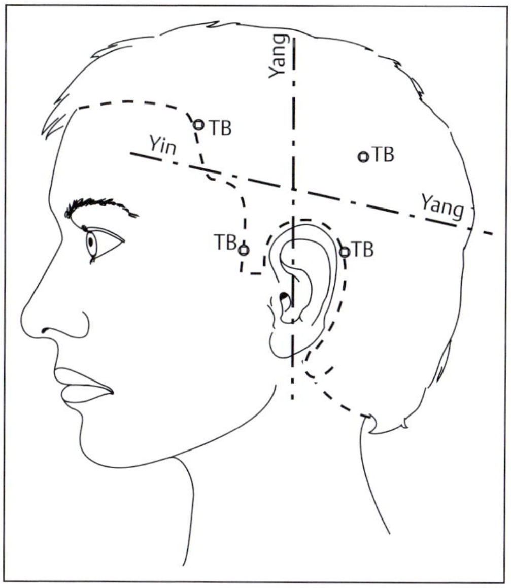

Figure 7–11 Ypsilon TB point.

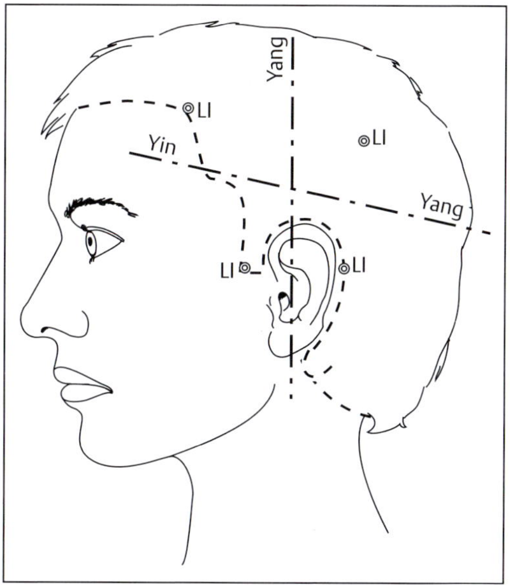

Figure 7–12 Ypsilon LI point.

Large Intestine (LI)

Yin of YIN Location: At the anterior hairline of the sideburn above the zygoma, see **Figure 7–12**.

Method of Location: With the patient seated and the physician standing in front and lateral to the patient, palpate just above the zygomatic process at the anterior aspect of the sideburn hairline, and palpate for a small hill.

咸 ䷞ 咸 ***Xián***

Mutual Influence—Lake Above, Mountain Below

"Sequence of the Gua: After Heaven
and Earth have come into existence,
there are myriad beings.
After myriad beings have come
into existence, there are male and female.
After male and female are distinguished,
there comes the relationship of
husband and wife.
After husband and wife have
united together, there arrive father
and son. After there are father and son,
there come ruler and minister.
After there are ruler and minister,
there come high and low.
After high and low exist,
then etiquette can be appropriately
practiced.
Decision
Mutual Influence.
Prosperous and smooth.
Favorable to be steadfast and upright.
Take a maiden as a wife.
Good fortune.
Lake on Mountain.
An image of Mutual Influence.
In correspondence with this,
The superior person opens his
heart and mind
To accept people without prejudice."[5]

References

Acupoint schema and charts are found on page 144 f.

1. Birch SJ, Felt RL. Understanding Acupuncture. London: Churchill Livingstone; 1999: 170–173
2. Ellis A, Wiseman N, Boss K. Fundamentals of Chinese Acupuncture. New York: Paradigm Publications; 1991: 29–31
3. Birch SJ, Felt RL. Understanding Acupuncture. London: Churchill Livingstone; 1999: 169–179
4. Feely R. Yamamoto new scalp acupuncture (YNSA) acupoint frequency in the treatment of herniated lumbar disk, lumbar radiculopathy, and mechanical low back pain. Medical Acupuncture 2005;16: 20–23
5. Huang A. The Complete I Ching. Rochester, VT: Inner Traditions; 1998: 264–267

8

YNSA Special Points

The Yellow Emperor asked Ch'i Po: "When the wind has harmed someone, it causes in some cases cold and heat… These illnesses are in each case different and [for this reason] carry different names. In some cases [the wind] penetrates deep into the body, to the five depots or the six palaces. The cause is unknown to me. I should therefore like to hear your explanations on this subject."

Ch'i Po: "When wind-influence is stored in the skin, it is unable to penetrate into the inner region [of the body] or to escape outside. The wind loves movement and makes its appearance in numerous variations. If wind-influence strikes the transportation [holes] of the five depots and six palaces, this also causes winds of the depots and palaces. Consequently, the wind is responsible for hundreds of different illnesses. Yet [in every case the illness is due] to the presence of wind-influences."[1]—Huang-di Nei-jing Su-wen

YNSA Special Points

There is a group of points that are related to Basic and Ypsilon points and are used for very specific medical diagnoses. They are tinnitus, aphasia, temporomandibular joint (TMJ) dysfunction, and female hormone dysfunction.

Tinnitus Points

Anatomical Correlate

Ipsilateral point: Tinnitus points consist of all four points taken together on the left and on the right. The four points used together are made up S-4 Yin of YIN and Yin of YANG plus two additional points between these two S-4 points.

Location

Yin of YIN: S-4 is located 0.7 cun below the hairline and 0.25 cun medial to the YIN C-1 line, see **Figure 8–1**. A little hill is palpated.

Yin of YANG: S-4 is located between the S-1 and S-2 points, medial to the YANG C-1 line. A little hill is palpated.

Yang of YIN: The YIN tinnitus point is located posterior to the Yin of YIN C-2 line (toes) ~0.5 cun anterior to a coronal line taken from the root of the pinna of the ear to the other ear, along an arc connecting the two S-4 points. It is not a little hill, but more of a depression.

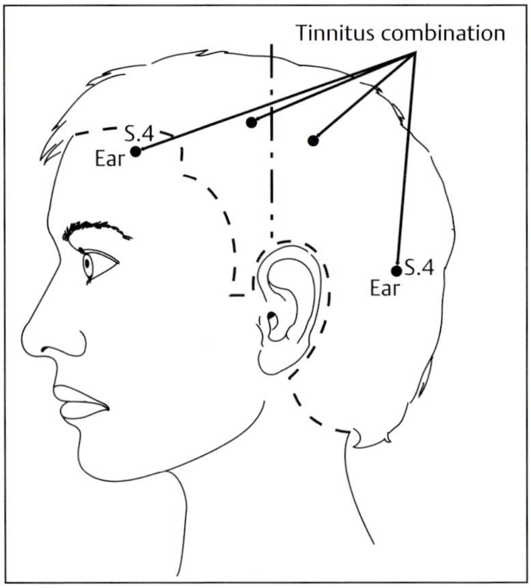

Figure 8–1 Tinnitus combination points.

Yang of YANG: The YANG tinnitus point is located ~1 cun posterior to a coronal line taken from the root of the pinna of one ear to the other ear, along an arc connecting the two S-4 points. It is not a little hill, but more of a depression. The point is ~3 mm in length.

Technique

Palpate each Tinnitus point and piqué subcutaneously at a 70 degree angle each point beginning at Yang of YANG and moving in order anteriorly ending with Yin of YIN.

Purpose and Use

The tinnitus points are used for vertigo, Ménière disease, and tinnitus.

Broca's Aphasia Point

Anatomical Correlate

Unilateral point: Broca's aphasia point is located over the temporal bone next to the right Yin of YIN KI Ypsilon point.

Location

It is located next to the KI Ypsilon point on the right, 1 to 3 mm anterior and inferior slightly down the KI point small hill of the temporal bone, see **Figure 8–2**. The aphasia point is about one-third of the way down the little hill of right-sided Yin of YIN KI point.

Technique

Palpate the right Yin of YIN KI Ypsilon point, move 1 to 3 mm anterior and inferior, sliding down the hill of the KI point, one-third of the way down. Piqué the point at a 70 degree angle.

Purpose and Use

The Broca's aphasia point is used for motor aphasia. The type of aphasia that is not fluent, slow,

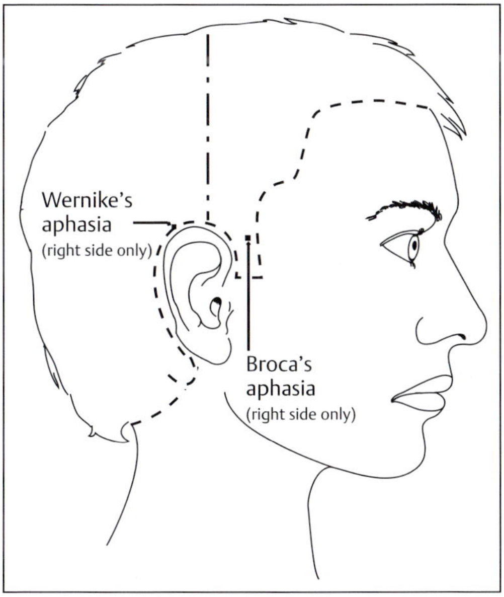

Figure 8–2 Aphasia points.

and laborious effort, with fair to good word and reading comprehension but impaired writing and repetition.

Wernicke's Aphasia Point

Anatomical Correlate

Unilateral point: Wernicke's aphasia point is located over the temporal bone next to the right Yang of YIN ST and SP Ypsilon points.

Location

It is located next to and between the ST and SP Ypsilon points on the right, see again **Figure 8–2**.

Technique

Palpate the right Yin of YANG SP, move superior 2 mm, and palpate for a small hill.

Purpose and Use

Wernicke's aphasia point is used for sensory aphasia. The type of aphasia with fluent, voluble speech that may be totally incomprehensible, with impaired word and reading comprehension, writing, and naming.

Temporomandibular Joint Point

Anatomical Correlate

Ipsilateral point: The TMJ point is located about halfway between the S-3 and S-4 points in both YIN and YANG.

Location

The TMJ point is on a little hill that is located on the frontal in YIN and occiput in YANG between these two points S-3 and S-4, see **Figure 8–3**.

Technique

Palpate S-3, move superior and laterally about one-half to two-thirds of the way toward S-4. Piqué at a 70 degree angle over the point or at a 20 degree angle to run the needle 10 to 15 mm subcutaneously between the S-3 and S-4 points.

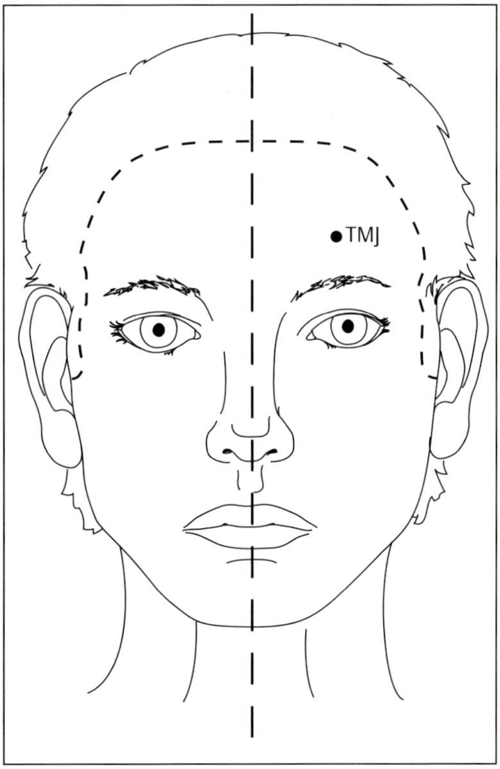

Figure 8–3 Temporomandibular joint point (Feely point).

Purpose and Use

TMJ dysfunction, dental, and facial pain.

Female Hormonal Z-S Point

Anatomical Correlate

Bilateral point: The Z-S point is located in the center of the following four points: lung, pericardium on the top, small intestine, and stomach on the bottom.

Location

The location is between these four points.

Technique

Palpate the Ypsilon lung point and move medially half way to the pericardium point and then move half way down to the second level (horizontal line) of points, that being small intestine and stomach. Piqué at 90 degree angle on the point. The Z-S point was discovered by Dorothea Zeise-Suess, M.D. in a retrospective clinical study of 271 women with hypermenorrhea, menometrorrhagia, secondary amenorrhea, and climacteric syndrome; 99% of the patients improved.[2]

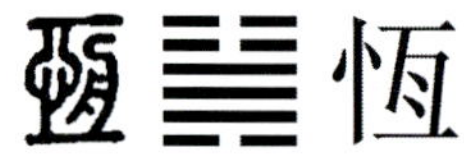

Héng

Long Lasting—Thunder Above, Wind Below

"Sequence of the Gua: The union of husband and wife should not be short-lived.
Thus, after Mutual Influence,
Long Lasting follows.
Decision
Long Lasting.
Prosperous and smooth.
No fault.
Favorable to be steadfast and upright.
Favorable to have somewhere to go.
The union of Thunder and Wind.
An image of Long Lasting.
In correspondence with this,
The superior person stands firm without changing his aim."[3]

References

Acupoint schema and charts are found on page 144 f.

1. Unschuld PU. Medicine in China: A History of Ideas. Berkeley: University of California Press; 1985: 273–275
2. Zeise-Suess D. New YNSA ZS Point for Disturbances of Female Hormonal Systems. Medical Acupuncture 2008(1):51–53
3. Huang A. The Complete I Ching. Rochester, VT: Inner Traditions; 1998: 272–274

From the Ling Shu: "The importance of the de qi *lies in the ability to feel the arrival of* qi. *The judgment of therapeutic effect depends on it. In the process of acupuncture, first watch for the approaching of qi to the point of* de qi. *If however, nothing arrives at the end of treatment, healing of disease is not to be expected." – Zhen Jiu Da Cheng*

"You can't expect both ends of a sugar cane to be sweet." – Chinese Proverb

9

Needling Techniques and Selection

Anatomy of an Acupoint

Professor Dr. Hartmut Heine, from the Institute für Antihomotoxikologie und Grundregulation in Baden-Baden, Germany, discovered the anatomical basis for acupuncture points (acupoints) in 1987 at the University of Witten, Herdecke, Germany. In the superficial body fascia, the corpus superficialis, there are collagenous layers separating the connective tissue of the skin and the muscles. The fascia corpus superficialis covers the entire body except the head, fingers, and toes. Near the acupuncture points, the fascia corpus superficialis is penetrated by a nerve-vessel bundle covered loosely with connective tissue. This nerve-vessel bundle is made up of arteriole capillaries, veins, venules, unmyelinated nerve fibers, and myelinated nerves with lymphatic vessels just above the superficial fascia. The acupoint is described as a vertical column, one could say a chimney, of loose connective tissue that is surrounded by the thick, dense connective tissue of the skin.[1] This perforation is present in the form of a laceration or a round opening. For this reason, there is a decrease in electrical resistance near the acupuncture point. Even in areas of the body where there is no superficial body fascia, such as the head, fingers, and toes, there are acupuncture points that can be demonstrated. These points are quite often sensitive. In the temporal region there is superficial temporal fascia, fatty tissue with veins and nerves over a deep sheath of temporal fascia. In other areas, going from superficial to deep, there is the superficial sheath of the temporal fascia followed by a deep sheath of temporal fascia, followed by the temporal artery with nerves. It is in this subcutaneous area below the deep sheath of the temporal fascia, and superior to the periosteum of the temporal bone, that one will place the acupuncture needle tip for effective YNSA treatment. This area of connective tissue houses nerves and vessels. It is from the selective bioelectrical stimulation with the acupuncture needle on these biocircuits of tissues, nerves, and vessels that physiological and biochemical changes are initiated.

Reichmamis in 1997 demonstrated electrical correlates of acupuncture points and documented the low resistance pathways for the flow of electricity along the acupuncture channels.[2] Yoshio Manaka in 1995 proposed the X-Signal System Theory. The X-Signal System represents a permanent regulatory system that is different from the classical nerves or hormonal system. This primitive sensory system is present in single-cell animals that did not have nerves per se but nevertheless reacted to external stimuli. The energy fields of the body and the perineural system, along with the living matrix, are some of the substrates through which the X-Signal System exerts its effects on the cells and tissues. Stimulation of the channel and its branches extends to every part of the body including the surfaces and interiors of each individual cell and organelle. Manaka theorized that through this primitive system one is able to influence all of the cells in the body through acupuncture. It is because the molecular web of the body is more than a mechanical anatomical structure; it is a continuous vibratory network and as such presents possibilities of great significance.[3] See also the discussion of the paper by Kenneth Pienta and Donald Coffrey on pages 46–47.

The Needle

A sterile, filiform non-cutting needle is the needle for performing acupuncture. It is generally made from stainless steel wire that is sharpened at one end. At the opposite end is a handle composed of thin, double-wound copper wire, stainless steel, silver, or molded piece of plastic. The needle has a point, which is described as bullet shaped, where the needle is used to push aside the horny plates of the epidermis, as opposed to cutting through the skin like a hypodermic or cutting (suturing) needle. The body of the needle is the part that is placed within the skin and scalp. At the end of the handle is a small tail where the copper or silver metal is wound in a double loop. Sterilized stainless steel needles are the best because of flexibility, strength, and resistance to oxidation.[4] The copper wire handle is preferred because it offers more electrical potential based on the physics of the two different metals—copper attached to stainless steel. Stainless steel, silver, or gold handles are energetically preferred over plastic.

Physics of the Needle

The physics of the copper-wound acupuncture needle has more than just electrical potential effects between the low resistance acupoint, the stainless needle conduction, and the difference between the copper and stainless steel electroscalar and magnetic vector potentials. Those two gradient potentials are usually enough to have a bioelectrical effect, as demonstrated with the ordinary stainless steel needles with either an annealed stainless steel or plastic handle, but the copper-wound needles possess other physical influences as demonstrated through the Aharonov-Bohm effect, a cornerstone of quantum mechanics.[5]

In classical physics, waves can interfere with each other. When two waves of the same frequency are in phase, their amplitudes add together to create larger waves; this is called constructive interference. When their waves are exactly out of phase, their amplitudes subtract and they can partially or completely cancel or destroy each other; this is called destructive interference. In nature, these interacting waves have a mix of frequency phases and therefore add and subtract in a very complex manner.

Wittaker and Tesla in 1904 generated potential waves and called them "non-hertzian waves."[2] When a magnetic field induces a current flow in a conductor, such as an acupuncture needle, it is actually the potential component of the field and not the field itself that underlies the effect. The potentials are of two types: scalar and magnetic vectors. Aharonov and Bohm in 1959 showed these potentials to have a physical reality.[6] A magnetic vector potential occurs when electrons pass through the force field region around a coil, as in a coiled copper-wound needle. Though there was no electricity, nevertheless these electrons undergo a phase change indicating that some nonelectric, nonmagnetic physical entity must be acting on it. Thus, the entity is called a magnetic vector potential.

Further research showed the existence of electric scalar potential in a region where no electric field existed. Thus, in destructive interference, where two electrical potentials cancel each other, electrostatic scalar potentials and magnetic vector potentials still remain. In essence, the energy and information contained in the original waves are not destroyed by interference.

Various kinds of coil designs enable the vectors of the electric and magnetic fields to destructively interfere or cancel each other out. The standard coil emits electric and magnetic fields in the space around it. The bifilar coil has the electric and magnetic fields cancelling each other out, thus producing electric scalar and magnetic vector fields. This bifilar coil is similar to the copper coil on copperwound acupuncture needles, which produces electric scalar and magnetic vector waves. According to Jacob and Rein, scalar waves appear to interact at atomic nuclei rather than with electrons. These interactions are described by quantum chromodynamics. Oschman states that scalar waves appear to be intimately involved in healing and are probably emitted by living systems.[2]

Needle Selection

Acupuncture needles used in YNSA are typically gauge 2, 3, 5, and, rarely, 8, see **Table 9–1**. The typical length is either 30 mm or 40 mm for gauge 2, 3, and 5; for gauge 8, 30 mm is sufficient. Gauge 5 followed by gauge 2 are the most commonly used in the author's YNSA experience. Gauge 8 0.30 mm needles are only used on very tightly restricted calcifications identified subcutaneously in the scalp or where a gauge 5 needle is not able to separate this calcification. A thin needle provides a less potent stimulus than a thicker needle but causes less pain. Gauge 2 is preferred for YNSA points on the forehead.

Presterilized disposable needles with tubes are ideally used in YNSA. As one places the finger of one hand over the point, one can with the other hand then slide the needle in the tube over the point, thus making sure one is exactly on the point with greater accuracy by using the tube. The use of the tube aids in getting the correct pre-

Table 9–1 Needle gauge table

Gauge (mm)	1 0.16	2 0.18	3 0.20	5 0.25	8 0.30
Length (mm)	30 40	30 40	30 40	30 40	30 –
Handle color	Red	Light blue	Dark blue	Purple	Brown

scribed depth for initial needle insertion, presenting the needle in a vertical position, ready to be adjusted to the correct angle as needed, in as sterile and clean a manner as possible through hair.

The constant controversy of what is the best (the thinnest, pain-free, but powerful) needle for one to use is the acupuncturist's elusive quest. The goal of the YNSA physician acupuncturist is to place the needle as painlessly as possible in the subcutaneous tissue to bioelectrically stimulate the body, thereby alleviating pain and restoring harmony and physiological balance. Often there are subcutaneous calcifications especially at the Basic point lines; for example, A-1–7, C-1, C-2, that require a stiff needle to be used to help separate the partially calcified subcutaneous tissue. However, using the thinnest needle offers the least amount of pain to the patient. Taking that into consideration, identifying the thinnest possible needle that does not bend and yet has a powerful effect is still the challenge.

Patient Position

The most common patient position is seated; occasionally they are supine or prone. For patients who suffer from a history of needle shock or fainting, a supine posture is recommended if YNSA is used at all, otherwise the patient is seated facing the physician.

Clean Needle Technique

Sterilizing the scalp is not done. Utilizing sterile single use disposable needles (preferably with an insertion tube) on a clean field is sufficient. Sterilizing the scalp can only be done with standard sterile procedures, which include shaving the head, followed by painting the scalp with 2% Iodine that may or may not be removed by isopropyl alcohol, and then properly draping the head to provide a sterile field. This, of course, is not done in YNSA.

In YNSA technique, when placing a sterile needle in the scalp, passing through the hair to get to the scalp, and keeping the needle sterile with or without a sterile tube is, for all intents and purposes, impossible. Simply using sterile needles on clean (recently washed) scalp and hair is acceptable; however, clean needle placement is recommended. “Clean needle technique” is defined by Jenny Belluomini as:

1. Wash hands before and after patient contact.
2. Swab the insertion site with alcoholized sterile gauze or sterile cotton ball. (Caution—Hair dyes and coloring may be altered with alcohol. Consult with patient before using.)
3. Keep needle shaft sterile (using a sterile tube) until it is inserted into the skin.
4. Use gloves if coming in contact with body fluids, which is unlikely in YNSA.[7]

A cotton ball with alcohol may be used to clean the area prior to needle insertion and after needle removal. Needle insertion is best done with sterilized single use disposable needles in a tube, but may also be done without a tube.

Remove one needle at a time, covering the site with a sterile alcohol swab. Then place all needles into the portable sharps container at the patient's bedside, appropriately discarding the sharps container and bodily fluid swabs in the hazardous waste for incineration.

Needle Insertion Techniques

Needle insertion is composed of five phases:

(1) insertion of the needle beneath the superficial layers of the skin, (2) correct needle angle insertion to threading of the needle or piqué the acupoint, (3) insertion or movement of the needle to the proper depth, (4) eliciting characteristic physiological sensation obtaining *de qi*, and then (5) finally, if needed, thrusting the needle slowly subcutaneously, breaking up calcified bands of subcutaneous tissue along the Basic point lines.

The single finger press technique is the preferred method for performing YNSA. The first step is to press with the thumbnail or the nail of the index finger of the left hand if the physician is right-handed, over the skin surface identifying the little mountain/hill of the Ypsilon point or the Basic point needing treatment. The second step is to alcohol swab the site. The third step for the no tube method is to hold the needle handle with the right thumb and forefinger, if using an insertion tube, hold the needle and the tube together at the tail of the needle. Holding the handle with the right index finger and thumb, guide the needle with or without a tube over the exact point where the left thumbnail has identified the proper acupoint. The fourth step is inserting the needle through the skin with a quick, firm downward motion or tap on the needle held in the tube. When palpating over an artery, use the pressing finger/thumb to cover the pulse, insert the needle next to it, protecting the blood vessel from injury during insertion.

Needle Angle and Depth of Insertion

The angle and depth are especially important in YNSA because the thickness of the scalp in the adult is only about 0.2 cun. The scalp is composed of five layers of skin: the hypodermis (which is the superficial fascia), the galeal aponeurotic, the muscle (occiput, frontal, temporal, etcetera), and the subaponeurotic and periosteum of the cranium. The first three layers are closely associated to each other and are difficult to separate. Ultimately the needle placement will be below these three layers and in the subaponeurotic space above the periosteum, see **Figure 9–1**.

The needling directions used in this text involve perpendicular, periperpendicularoblique, transverse oblique, and transverse insertions; see **Figure 9–2**. Perpendicular denotes a 90 degree angle to the skin's surface. Periperpendicular-oblique denotes an angle of approximately 70 degrees to the skin's surface. Transverse oblique denotes an angle of approximately 15 to 20 degrees to the skin's surface. Transverse denotes an insertion parallel to the skin's surface through the subcutaneous tissue after the dermal layer has been penetrated. It is important to note that the needling directions are always relative to the skin's surface and the contour of the skull rather than to absolute horizontal.

Ypsilon points are usually treated using a perpendicular or a periperpendicular insertion. For most Basic points where the needle is taking in several segments of the point or a line of points, such as A-1–7 or D-1–6, the needle is started in a transverse oblique position of 15 to 20 degrees. Then, after the needle has penetrated the skin into the subaponeurotic space, it is changed to a transverse position and the needle is further inserted parallel to the periosteum, sliding along in the subaponeurotic space, putting the body of the needle through the hard calcifications and ridges that are imposing upon the subaponeurotic space. The needle should be inserted just over the desired area but not so deep as to have the handle of the needle above the insertion hole. After the needle has opened the subaponeurotic space, usually tonification is performed by twisting (clockwise rotation) the handle between the thumb and index finger for less than 360 degrees.

Needling Manipulation Techniques

The needle is left in place for 15 to 20 minutes and slowly withdrawn by pressing the skin around the point with the thumb and index finger, slightly rotating the needle gently, and lifting it slowly to the subcutaneous level and then withdrawing the needle quickly. Follow that by pressing the acupuncture point with your gloved finger or, if necessary, with a cotton ball to prevent bleeding.

The techniques for needle manipulation include lifting and thrusting, twirling and rotating, and retaining the needle. Most Ypsilon points use retaining the needle and occasionally twirling and rotating. Most Basic points use retaining the needle, twirling, and rotating with lifting and thrusting only over lines (A-1–7, C-2, E-1–12, etcetera) with firm calcification identified.

The needle manipulation of lifting and thrusting occurs after the *de qi* has been obtained; the needle is pulled out a short distance and then thrust back in subcutaneously. This is typically done in treating lines A-1–7 or C-2, breaking up the calcifications subcutaneously, and rarely on C-1. The usual distance of this motion is half the needle length, <15 mm. Slow movements are tonifying while fast movements are more draining and dispersing.

Twirling and rotating occur when the needle is inserted and *de qi* is obtained. Then one would grasp the needle between the thumb and forefinger and twist the needle, but not exceeding 360 degrees. Rotating the needle rapidly in a wide arc is a dispersing method and is less frequently done. Using a slower motion and lesser arc pro-

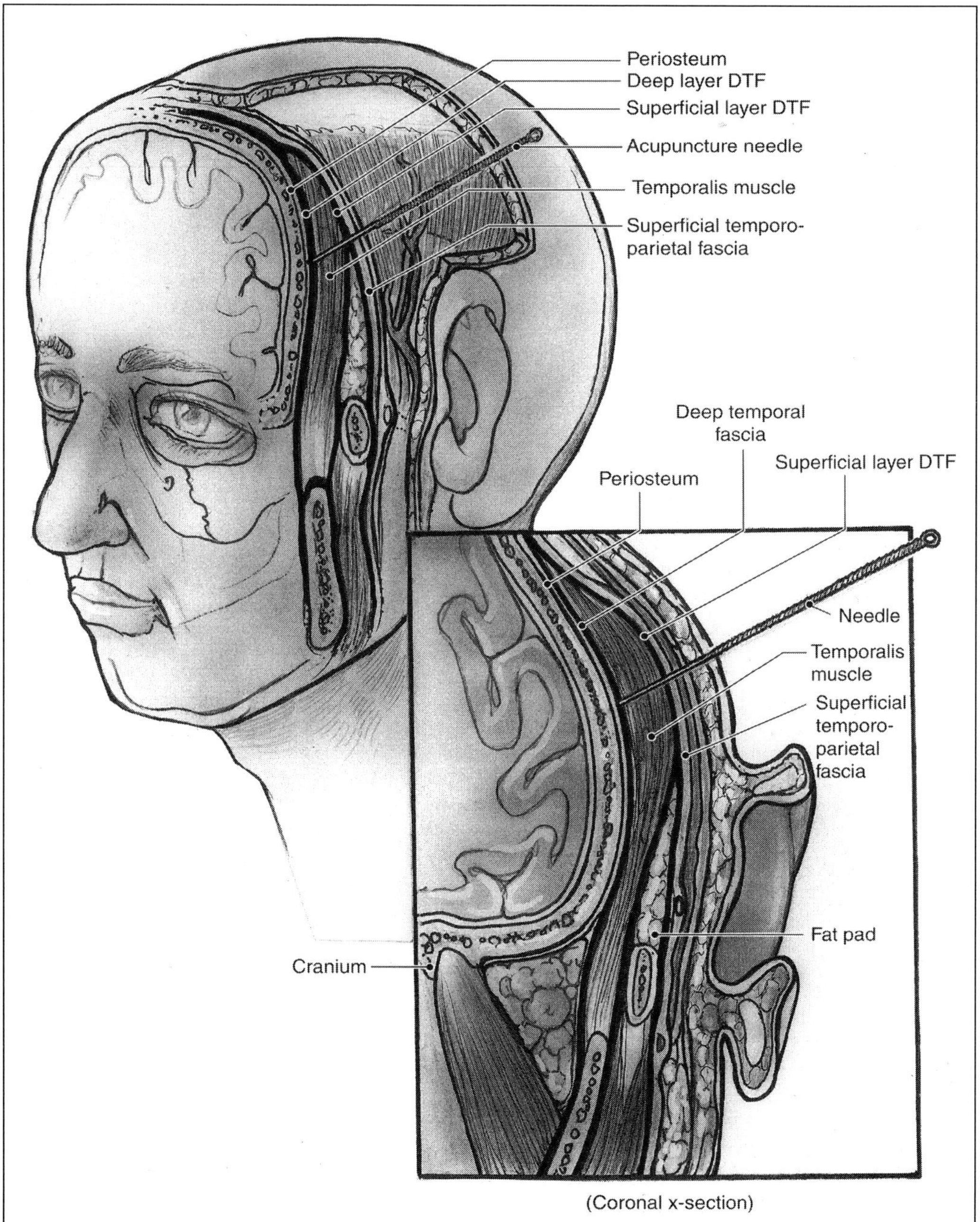

Figure 9–1 Scalp layers and depth of needle insertion.

vides stimulation and tonification. This twirling method is most commonly used in the Basic point D-1–6 and in the Ypsilon points.

Retaining the needle is the way most YNSA is practiced. This includes placing the needle in the proper position, usually obtaining *de qi*. Needle retention, in general, can increase the ability of the point to relieve pain and quiet the spirit. Most retention is between 15 and 20 minutes for tonification and 40 minutes for dispersion. Most

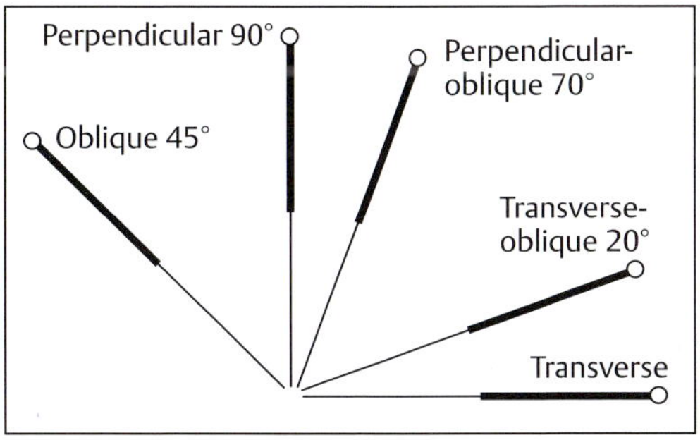

Figure 9–2 Needling angles.

cases in the author's experience require tonification and not dispersion.

Course of Treatment

In the case of chronic diseases, in Japan it is not uncommon to treat the patient every day for a course of 10 to 20 treatments. In acute cases, the course of treatment may be varied from 1 to 10 treatments. In the United States, it is common to treat chronic cases on an outpatient basis once or twice a week, and daily as a patient in a hospital or residential pain center.

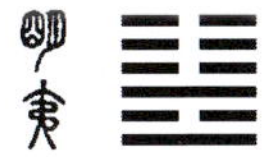 明夷 ***Míng yí***

Brilliance Injured—Earth Above, Fire Below

"Sequence of the Gua: Proceeding Forward without restraint, surely someone will be hurt. Thus, after Proceeding Forward, Brilliance Injured follows.
Decision
Brilliance Injured.
Favorable to be steadfast and upright in hardship.
Brightness has sunk under the Earth.
An image of Brilliance Injured.
In correspondence with this,
The superior person remains in harmony with the multitude.
Covering his brilliance,
yet his light is still shining."[7]

References

Additional references are available on page 148.

1. Helms J. Acupuncture Energetics: A Clinical Approach for Physicians. Berkeley: Medical Acupuncture Publishers; 1995: 26
2. Oschman JL. Energy Medicine: the scientific basis. Edinburgh: Churchill Livingstone; 2000: 69
3. Oschman JL. Energy Medicine: The Scientific Basis. Edinburgh, UK: Churchill Livingstone; 2000: 69–72,206
4. Birch SJ, Felt RL. Understanding Acupuncture. London: Churchill Livingstone; 1999: 261
5. Aharonov Y, Bohm D. Significance of electromagnetic potentials in the quantum theory. Phys Rev (Ser. 2) 1959;115: 485–491
6. Belluomini J. Clean Needle Technique: A Manual for Acupuncturists and Other Healthcare Professionals. Brookline, MA: Complementary Medicine Press; 1999: 69–70
7. Huang A. The Complete I Ching. Rochester, VT: Inner Traditions; 1998: 299–301

10

YNSA Treatment Protocols

"The stability of the inner environment is a cardinal requirement for the preservation of well being."[1]

"There is no wave without the wind." – Chinese Proverb

Principles of Treatment

My osteopathic family practice director said, "More mistakes in medicine are made by not looking, than by not knowing." The same holds true in acupuncture. The recommended treatment protocol is determined after one has done a history and physical examination, made a medical diagnosis, made an acupuncture/Oriental Medicine diagnosis, and have determined with the patient that acupuncture is indicated and acceptable because it could be helpful. One then starts refining the YNSA diagnosis and first begins the treatment phase with YNSA Basic points.

Finding the Basic and Ypsilon points is difficult at first. This psychomotor skill, as well as YNSA needling techniques, is best learned one-on-one with an expert instructor. The companion DVD included with this book will be helpful for learning, modeling, and practicing. The Basic and Ypsilon points are always little ridges, mountains, or palpable hills in the scalp as one searches the scalp with the palpatory thumb or finger. Treat the anatomical correlate ipsilateral to the pain, dysfunction, or disease. Determine sidedness for neck diagnosis, use the procedure depicted in **Figures 5–1**, **5–2**, and **5–3** in Chapter 5. Use YNSA neck diagnosis whenever possible to confirm need for treatment. Retest the neck diagnosis after needle placement in the scalp to ascertain correct needle placement. If still positive, reposition the needle until the neck diagnosis is improved. If YNSA neck diagnosis is not possible, use YNSA abdominal diagnosis or TCM/Five Phase pulse diagnosis.

In neuromusculoskeletal conditions and somatic problems, treat first with Basic points in the appropriate phase YIN or quadrants based on the above decisions. Palpate the neck diagnosis Basic points (lumbar spine, thoracic spine, cervical spine, brain) first for tenderness. If tenderness is present, piqué the corresponding YNSA Basic point. To find the point, consult the figure or bedside chart, palpate for a small mountain or hill, press with your fingernail to elicit tenderness if unsure of the exact location on the scalp. Positive YNSA points are also tender to deep pressure.

Basic points such as A-1–7, C-1, C-2, and D-1–6 are piqued transverse-oblique at a 20 degree angle to thread the needle subcutaneously. Points S-1, S-2, S-3, and S-4 are piqued periperpendicularoblique at a 45 degree angle. All other Basic points are piqued perpendicular-oblique at a 70 degree angle. YNSA points are piqued perpendicular at a 90 degree angle.

YNSA Protocol Rules

The basic rules regarding the protocols listed below are few and simple. (1) Only treat what is absolutely needed to achieve a positive effect. (2) Using the listed points first will achieve a positive effect in most cases (see Chapter 12). (3) Ypsilon points are usually the key in getting 100% relief, especially in old and/or complicated conditions. (4) Follow the Ypsilon procedures in diagnosis and treatment. (5) Finally, Basic points work very well in acute cases and often are all that is needed.

Treating Pain

The general protocols for all painful conditions are to make the most specific diagnosis you can and determine the most probable causative factors and pathology present. Treat the condition medically and/or surgically first, as appropriate. Then treat with YNSA using the Basic points related to the anatomy that has or is causing the pain; for example, a painful finger. Treat ipsilaterally distally only C-1 (finger) and then if pain continues treat points A-4–7 over the correct spinal nerve root affecting the finger (C4–5, 5–6, or 6–7).

After the Basic points are treated, if pain persists, check YNSA Ypsilon neck diagnosis and treat any positive Ypsilon points. If pain persists, move on to check abdominal diagnosis and treat positive findings using Basic and/or Ypsilon points. If pain still persists, make a TCM/Five Phase radial pulse diagnosis and treat positive findings based on channel diagnosis; for example, with a weak LR pulse, treat YNSA Ypsilon LR point left in the correct quadrant.

Remember, pain is a subjective symptom; you must be a physician and use all of your clinical, medical, and surgical skills, since YNSA is a powerful tool but not a panacea.

 ䷚ 益 *Yi*

Nourishing—Mountain Above, Thunder Below

"Sequence of the Gua:
When things are accumulated
in great amount, nourishing becomes
available. Thus, after Great Accumulation,
Nourishing follows.
Decision
Nourishing.
Being steadfast and upright: good fortune.
Watch your nourishment;
Pay attention to what is in your mouth.
Thunder beneath Mountain.
An image of Nourishing.
In correspondence with this,
The superior person is careful
of his words
And moderate in eating and drinking."[2]

References

Additional references are available on page 148.

1. Unschuld PU. Medicine in China: A History of Ideas. Berkeley: University of California Press; 1985: 355
2. Huang A. The Complete I Ching. Rochester, VT: Inner Traditions; 1998: 234–236

11

YNSA Treatment Protocol and Practical Procedures

The Yellow Emperor asked Shao-shih: "I have heard it said that the existence of man encompasses firmness and softness, weakness and strength, short and long duration, as well as yin *and* yang *[regions]. I should like to discover in what relationship all this stands to the methods [of therapy]."*

Ch'i Po: "In yin *there is* yang*, in* yang *there is* yin*. When one is knowledgeable about* yin *and* yang*, he can apply needle treatments methodically. When the origins of illness have been comprehended, the application of needles can be carried out on the basis of the [proper] principles. Carefully assess the causes of the affliction … Therefore it is said that when the illness is located in the yin-in-yin [region], apply needles to the brook transportation [points] of the* yin *[channels]. If the illness is located in the yang-in-yang [region], apply needles to the confluence [points] of the* yang *[channels]. If the illness is located in the yin-in-yang [sphere], apply needles to the stream [points] of the* yin *[channels]. If the illness is located in the yang-in-yin [sphere], apply needles to the network [channels]."[1]—Huang-di Nei-jing Su-wen*

Practice Guidelines

The following are a list of straightforward office guidelines that the author has used over the years, having assimilated and mastered Dr. Yamamoto's YNSA technique.

1. Always make your medical diagnosis first.
2. Then decide if YNSA is indicated on this patient today by history, physical exam, and patient's receptivity to acupuncture.
3. Next, formulate an Oriental Medical diagnosis; this could be Traditional Chinese Medicine (TCM), Eight Principle, Five Phase, or YNSA Neck Diagnosis.
4. Formulate the main goal of your treatment; for example, pain relief to the left arm and shoulder, or balance Five Phase (pulse diagnosis).
5. Do other procedures before YNSA, such as manipulation, prescriptions, counseling, or other TCM, Energetics body acupuncture, but leave various pharmaceutical, trigger point, or nutraceutical injections to the very end of the visit, after YNSA.
6. Palpate the LI-4, *he gu,* point to determine which side is most tender. If you can not tell the difference with the patient's help, then palpate both left and right liver (LR) neck diagnostic points simultaneously, to see which one is most tender. If you still can not tell which is most tender, then go to the kidney (KI) neck diagnostic point left and right, palpating simultaneously to see which one is tender. If you still can not tell, go to the YNSA abdominal diagnosis techniques. If you still can not tell, do TCM or Five Phase radial pulse diagnosis.
7. Palpate the liver (LR) YNSA neck diagnosis point on the tender side to determine if the sternocleidomastoid muscle (SCM) is hard or soft. If the SCM is soft, treat in YANG and if firm, treat in YIN. About 90% of the time, it is hard/firm, so you treat in the YIN phase. The remaining 10% of the time it is soft, therefore you treat in YANG.
8. Treat Basic points first. Palpate for tenderness and find the little mountain/hill associated with the Basic point that the history and physical examination indicate needs to be treated.
9. Have your acupuncture needles very close to you as you palpate with one hand using a single finger or thumb, indent the scalp soft tissue with that thumbnail or fingernail. Then with needle in hand, place the needle at the correct marked spot at the desired angle to achieve its greatest effect.
10. Follow the YNSA Basic point treatment protocol. When finished, move on to perform the YNSA neck and/or YNSA abdomen and/or TCM radial pulse diagnosis. The YNSA neck diagnosis is preferred to see if tenderness is gone, verifying proper needle placement.
11. Next, follow the YNSA treatment protocol in this book as needed.
12. Piqué the most tender Ypsilon point on the most tender side first. Continue treating all positive Ypsilon points until the LI-4, *he gu,* point is no longer tender on both sides. At that point you are finished and the patient will have maximum pain relief and a harmonically balanced electromagnetic field as demonstrated by the Oriental Medicine pulse diagnosis, if done correctly.
13. Have the patient lie down and rest while the needles do their work for ~20 minutes.
14. Remove the needles, do any other pharmaceutical or nutraceutical injections, although quite often trigger points are no longer needed, and discharge the patient for that day with standard acupuncture precautions listed below.

Acupuncture Precautions

Standard acupuncture precautions as used in powerful French Energetic or Five Phase spirit treatments are not always required but are routinely used. They are especially helpful with first time and extensive YNSA treatments. For the 24 hours following the YNSA treatment, and especially for the first 12 hours, the precautions are:

- No heavy exercise
- No large and/or heavy meals
- No alcohol
- No sex

Documentation

Finally, on page 146 f. is a standard YNSA acupuncture/musculoskeletal progress note that may be copied and used to facilitate uniformity of care and improve documentation.

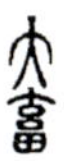 ䷙ 大畜 ***Dà chù***

Great Accumulation—Mountain Above, Heaven Below

"Sequence of the Gua: When truthfulness is present, accumulation is possible. Thus, after Without Falsehood, Great Accumulation follows. Decision Great Accumulation. Favorable to be steadfast and upright. Eat not at home. Good fortune. Favorable to cross great rivers. Heaven between Mountains. An image of Great Accumulation. In correspondence with this, The superior person has a wide learning And memory of the words and deeds of the past, In order to accumulate his virtue."[2]

References

Additional references are available on page 148. Acupoint schema and charts are found on page 144 f.

1. Unschuld PU. Medicine in China: A History of Ideas. Berkeley: University of California Press; 1985: 269–270
2. Huang A. The Complete I Ching. Rochester, VT: Inner Traditions; 1998: 227–229

12

YNSA Treatment

Zhen Jiu Jia Yi Jing says: "The superior physician controls disease before any illness has declared itself; the average practioner uses acupuncture before the disease has come to its crisis; the inferior practitioner treats the patient when the illness is already dying away."[1]

In this chapter, some of the more common medical diagnoses and protocols for treating them using YNSA are discussed.

A listing of anatomical sites and the corresponding channels that could be disturbed when pathology is located there is given in **Table 12–1** and the Seven Emotions and their related channels are listed in **Table 12–2**. Please use this treatment point list as a guide in selecting the proper Basic and Ypsilon points. Use the guide, in sequence, until one of two things happens, YNSA Neck/Abdominal Diagnosis or TCM/Five Phase Pulse Diagnosis is negative and symptoms improve. As always, one must rely on positive patient history, physical examination, and YNSA neck, YNSA abdominal, and/or TCM/Five Phase pulse diagnosis for final selection of all YNSA points to be used in the patient.

Table 12–1 Ypsilon and Basic points in order of importance based on TCM channel influence

Pain Site/Pathology	Ypsilon Points	Basic Points
Vertex of head	BL, LR, TB, GB	M-1, M-2
Brain	BL, ST	M-1, M-2, M-3
Forehead	ST, BL, LR, GB, TB, KI, SP, HT, SI	M-1, M-2
Face	LR, GB, BL, SI, TB, ST, LU, BL	M-2, S-1, S-2, S-3, S-4, TMJ
Eye	LR, HT, ST, GB, BL, SI, TB	M-2, S-1
Eyelid	Upper BL; Lower ST	M-2, S-1
Nose	ST, BL, LU, LI, ST, SI, LR	M-2, S-2
Maxillary/face	BL, ST, LI, SI	M-2, S-2, S-3
Submandibular	ST, GB, SI, TB, LI	M-2, S-2, S-3
Angle of the jaw	GB, ST	M-2, S-3, TMJ
Lips and mouth	ST, LR, LI, ST	S-3, TMJ
Teeth	LI, ST	S-3, TMJ
Tongue	TB, BL, HT, SP, KI	S-3
Ear	BL, GB, ST, SI, TB, LI, PC, KI, HT, LU, SP	M-2, S-4
Occipital region	BL, GB, KI	M-2, M-3
Pharynx and upper esophagus	SI, HT, GB, ST, SP, LI, BL	M-2, S-3, A-1–8
Trachea	ST, GB, LR, HT, PC, LI, LU	M-2, S-3, A-1–8
Epiglottis	LR	M-2, A-1–8
Larynx	KI	M-2, A-1–8
Nape of the neck	BL, SI, GB, KI, LI	A-1–8
Shoulder and scapula	BL, GB, SI, LI, TB, LU	A-1–8, C-1, B-1
Chest	HT, LU, PC, TB	E-1–12
Center of chest	LU, LI, HT, KI, LR	E-1–12

Table 12–1 (continued)

Pain Site/Pathology	Ypsilon Points	Basic Points
Heart	HT, SI, SP, KI, BL, GB, ST, TB	E-1–6, M-2, A-1–8
Pericardium	PC, TB, KI	E-1–6, A-1–8
Breast	ST, LI, GB, HT, ST	E-1–6
Spine	BL, KI, ST LI	A-1–8, E-1–12, D-1–6, D
Axilla	GB, LU HT, PC, SI, BL	B-1, C-1
Ribs and lateral costal region	GB, PC, LR, ST, LU, SP	E-1–12
Liver	LR, GB	E-6–12
Gall bladder	GB, LR	E-6–12
Lower back	BL, GB	D-1–6, D
Kidney	KI, BL	E-6–12
Buttocks	BL	F-1, D-1–6, C-2
Sacrococcyx	GB, BL	F-1, D-1–6, C-2
Abdomen	ST, SP, LR, KI, LI	E-6–12
Umbilicus	ST, SP, HT	E-6–12
Spleen	SP, ST	E-6–12
Stomach	ST, SP, SI, LR, LU	E-6–12
Intestines	LI, LU, SP, SI, HT	E-6–12, D-1–4
Bladder	BL, KI, TB	E-6–12, D-1–4
Triple burner	TB, PC, LU	E-1–12
Genital region	LR, ST, SP, KI	D-1–6
Hip	GB, LR, SP, ST, BL, KI	F1, D-1–6, C-2
Ankle, foot lateral	GB, BL, ST	C-2
Ankle, foot medial	KI, LR, SP	C-2
Knee lateral	GB, ST, BL	C-2, G-1
Knee medial	LR, SP, KI	C-2, G-3
Elbow lateral	LI, SI, TB	C-1
Elbow medial	HT, LU, PC	C-1
Hand/fingers lateral	SI, LU, TB	C-1
Hand/fingers medial	LI, HT, PC	C-1

Table 12–2 Seven emotions and related channels

Emotion	Channels
Joy	HT, PC
Anger	LR, GB, KI, HT
Anxiety	LU, SP
Work/concentration	SP, LU
Grief/sorrow	PC, LU, HT, LR
Fear	KI, HT
Fright	HT, KI

Protocols for Various Medical Diagnoses

Aphasia

1. Treat Basic point S-3.
2. Treat Aphasia special point for Broca's or Wernick's right side only.
3. Treat all positive Ypsilon points. Frequent points include HT, SI, KI, and BL.
4. Treat Basic points M-2, M-3.

Asnomia

1. Treat Basic points S-2.
2. Treat all positive Ypsilon points. Frequent points include LU, LI, ST, and SP.
3. Treat Basic points M-2, M-3.

Cervical Herniated Disks

1. Treat Basic points A-1–7.
2. Treat all positive Ypsilon points. Frequent points include GB, KI, PC, and BL.
3. Treat Basic points M-1, M-2, M-3.

Cervical Radiculopathy

1. Treat Basic points A-1–7 and Darm as needed for the specific nerve root involved ipsilaterally.
2. Treat Basic points C-1 ipsilaterally.
3. Treat Basic points M-2 and M-3 ipsilaterally.
4. Treat all positive Ypsilon points. Frequent points include GB, BL, KI, TB, ST, SP.
5. Treat all Basic points above bilaterally.

Cervicalgia

1. Treat Basic points A-1–7 ipsilaterally.
2. Treat all positive Ypsilon points. Frequent points include GB, BL, KI, SI, LI, ST.
3. Treat all Basic points above bilaterally.

Dental/Oral Pain

1. Treat S-3 ipsilaterally.
2. Treat Basic points A-1–7 ipsilaterally.
3. Treat all positive Ypsilon points. Frequent points include ST, SP, LI, LU, HT.
4. Treat TMJ point if indicated.
5. Treat all Basic points above bilaterally.

Ear Pain

1. Treat S-4 ipsilaterally.
2. Treat Basic points A-1–7 ipsilaterally.
3. Treat all positive Ypsilon points. Frequent points include KI, BL.

Entrapment Neuropathies

1. Treat Basic points related to entrapment neuropathy (M-1, M-2, and M-3) ipsilaterally.
2. Treat all positive Ypsilon points. Frequent points include KI, BL, PC, TB, GB, and LR.

Eye Pain—Conjunctivitis

1. Treat S-1 ipsilaterally.
2. Treat Basic points A-1–7 ipsilaterally.
3. Treat all positive Ypsilon points. Frequent points include LR, PC.

Facial Paralysis

1. Treat Basic points A-1–7, M-1, M-2, M-3 ipsilaterally.
2. Treat all positive Ypsilon points. Frequent points include ST, SP, LI, LU, HT, BL, GB, and KI.
3. Treat all Basic points above bilaterally.

Headaches

1. Treat Basic points M-1, M-2, M-3 ipsilaterally.
2. Treat Basic points A-1–7 ipsilaterally if suboccipital pain is present.
3. Treat all positive Ypsilon points. Frequent points include GB, LR, BL, TB, PC, ST, SI.
4. Treat all Basic points above bilaterally.

Hemiplegia

1. Treat Basic points M-2, M-3, M-1 bilaterally.
2. Treat affected anatomical part Basic points ipsilaterally for example, C-1 and C-2.
3. Treat all positive Ypsilon points. Frequent points include KI, SP, GB, LR, PC, HT.
4. Treat Basic point D and points D-1–6 bilaterally.
5. Treat Basic points A-1–7 bilaterally.
6. Treat Basic points E-1–12 bilaterally.

Lower Motor Neuron Lesions

1. Treat Basic points D-1–6, E-1–8 ipsilaterally.
2. Treat Basic points for all affected anatomical parts E, G-1, G-2, G-3, C-1, C-2 ipsilaterally.
3. Treat all positive Ypsilon points. Frequent points include KI, BL, GB, LR, PC, TB, and HT.
4. Treat all Basic points above bilaterally.

Lumbago/Low Back Pain

1. Treat Basic points D and/or D-1–6 ipsilaterally.
2. Treat all positive Ypsilon points. Frequent points include GB, BL, KI, SP, ST, MH, PC.
3. Treat all Basic points above bilaterally.

Lumbar Herniated Discs

1. Treat Basic points D-1–6 ipsilaterally.
2. Treat Basic points A-1–7.
3. Treat all positive Ypsilon points. Frequent points include GB, KI, and PC.
4. Treat C-2 and M-1.
5. Treat all Basic points above bilaterally.

Lumbar Radiculopathy

1. Treat Basic points D, and D-1–6, as needed for the specific nerve root involved ipsilaterally.
2. Treat Basic points C-2 ipsilaterally.
3. Treat Basic points D ipsilaterally.
4. Treat Basic point F.
5. Treat all positive Ypsilon points. Frequent points include GB, TB, BL, KI, SP, ST.
6. Treat all Basic points above bilaterally.

Paraplegia

1. Treat Basic points M-2, M-3, M-1 bilaterally.
2. Treat affected anatomical part Basic points bilaterally for example, C-2.
3. Treat all positive Ypsilon points. Frequent points include BL, GB, LR, KI, SP, PC, TB.
4. Treat Basic points D and D-1–6 bilaterally.
5. Treat Basic points A-1–7 bilaterally.
6. Treat Basic points E-1–12 bilaterally.

Sciatica

1. Treat Basic point F ipsilaterally.
2. Treat Basic points D and/or D-1–6 ipsilaterally.
3. Treat all positive Ypsilon points. Frequent points include GB, BL, KI, TB, PC, SP.
4. Treat all Basic points above bilaterally.

Sinusitis

1. Treat Basic points S-2, S-3, S-1 ipsilaterally.
2. Treat Basic points A-1–7 bilaterally.
3. Treat Basic points M-2, M-3.
4. Treat all positive Ypsilon points. Frequent points include SP, ST, LU, LI.

Stroke (CVA)

1. Treat Basic points M-2, M-3, M-1 bilaterally.
2. Treat affected anatomical part Basic points ipsilaterally.
3. Treat all positive Ypsilon points. Frequent points include KI, SP, GB, LR, PC, HT.

Thoracic Back Pain

1. Treat Basic points E-1–12 ipsilaterally.
2. Treat all positive Ypsilon points. Frequent points include BL, KI, ST, LI, GB, LR.
3. Treat all Basic points above bilaterally.
4. Treat Basic points A and D, D-1–6 if related to cervical and lumbar dysfunction or pathology.

Thoracic Herniated Disks

1. Treat Basic points E.
2. Treat Basic points A-1–7.
3. Treat all positive Ypsilon points. Frequent points include GB, KI, PC, TB, and BL.
4. Treat Basic points bilaterally.

Tinnitus

1. Treat tinnitus special points.
2. Treat all positive Ypsilon points. Frequent points include KI, BL, GB, PC.

Trigeminal Neuralgia

1. Treat Basic points M-1, M-2, M-3.
2. Treat Basic points A-1–7.
3. Treat all positive Ypsilon points. Frequent points include ST, SP, LI, LU, GB, and BL.

Upper Extremity Pain

1. Treat Basic point C-1.
2. Treat Basic points B-1, A-1–7.
3. Treat all positive Ypsilon points. Frequent points include LI, SI, HT, LU, TB, PC.

鼎 ䷱ 鼎 ***Dǐng***

Establishing the New—Fire Above, Wind Below

Sequence of the Gua: "For changing things absolutely, there is nothing better than a ding. Thus, after Abolishing the Old, Establishing the New follows. Decision Establishing the New. Supreme good fortune. Prosperous and smooth. Fire over Wood. An image of Establishing the New. In correspondence with this, The superior person rectifies his position And fulfills the will of Heaven."[1]

References

Additional references are available on page 148. Acupoint schema and charts are found on page 144f.

1. Huang A. The Complete I Ching. Rochester, VT: Inner Traditions; 1998: 397–399

13

Case Reports

"In the ancient times
The sages worked on I.
They followed the truth of nature
And the meaning of destiny.
They established the Tao of Heaven
And named it yin and yang.
They established the Tao of Earth
And named it yielding and firm.
They established the Tao of Humanity
And named it benevolence and justice.
They combined these three and doubled them.
Therefore, in I, six yao [lines] make up an accomplished gua [six line symbols].
They differentiated yao into yin and yang,
Now by the yielding and now by the firm.
Thus, in I, a system of six places was formed."[1]—
I Ching

The following is a collection of 18 reports to demonstrate how YNSA is easily integrated into cranial osteopathic manipulation practice. These neuromusculoskeletal cases are typical of YNSA's usefulness and effectiveness in medical practice.

Cervical Herniated Disk/Cervical Radiculopathy

Chief Complaint
Neck and thumb pain.

History
46-year-old female with neck and shoulder pain for the past 3 months. Numbness and tingling of the right first two fingers and in the arm. MRI shows a herniated disc at C5–C6 with pinching on the thecal sac.

Key Physical Findings
Deep tendon reflexes were +2/+2 biceps and triceps. Sensation diminished with numbness of the right index finger and thumb. Somatic dysfunction was found with C2–C4 rotated left sidebent left, C5–C6 rotated right sidebent right, T4–T7 rotated left sidebent right, L5 rotated left sidebent left, anterior right innominate, left sacral torsion.

Diagnosis
Cervical radiculopathy with herniated nucleus pulposus C5–C6, somatic dysfunction of the head, cervical, thoracic, lumbar, sacrum, and pelvis, and myositis.

Treatment Type
Osteopathic manipulation using indirect, myofascial release, articulatory, and high velocity/low amplitude techniques, and YNSA.

Frequency: One visit.

Details: Yin of YIN right M-2, A, B-1, and C-1.

Response
100% pain relief of thumb and index finger numbness and arm pain.

Cervical Radiculopathy

Chief Complaint
Constant burning and pain in the neck and shoulder that started 1 week prior. Numbness in the left distal index finger radiating from the neck into the left shoulder blade, and tingling of the left arm. Pain is 2/10.

History
59-year-old female hairdresser with chronic neck, shoulder, and arm pain. She has had two motor vehicle accidents within the last 9 months.

Key Physical Findings
Deep tendon reflexes +2/+4 equal bilateral. C2 rotated left sidebent left, C1 rotated left, C6 rotated right sidebent right, C4–C7 rotated right sidebent left, L5 rotated right sidebent left, left sacral torsion, and anterior right innominate.

Diagnosis
Cervical radiculopathy, post-traumatic acceleration/deceleration injury/whiplash, myositis, and somatic dysfunction of the head, cervical, thoracic, lumbar, sacrum, and pelvis.

Treatment Type
Osteopathic manipulation using indirect, myofascial release techniques and YNSA.

Frequency: Patient received weekly treatments for 6 weeks.

Details: The left Yin of YIN PC, SP, KI, and BL. Right Yin of YIN KI. Left Yin A, D-1–6. A diagnosis of spinal stenosis and bulging cervical discs was made with subsequent MRIs. Pain continued to be modulated with YNSA acupuncture and gradually diminished with no surgeries performed.

Response
100% pain relief.

Chronic Cervicalgia

Chief Complaint
Cervicalgia with burning sensation into the hands from the neck.

History
Pain for the past 2 years.

Key Physical Findings
Areas of somatic dysfunction of the head, cervical, thoracic, lumbar, sacrum, and pelvis.

Diagnosis
Somatic dysfunction of the head, cervical, thoracic, lumbar, sacrum, and pelvis; neuritis; and cervicalgia.

Treatment Type
Osteopathic manipulation using indirect, high velocity/low amplitude, articulatory procedures and YNSA.

Frequency: Monthly visits.

Details: YNSA left Yin of YIN HT, SI, and KI. Yin left and right M-2, M-3, and A.

Response
100 % pain relief post-treatment.

Chronic Migraine

Chief Complaint
Migraine headaches.

History
Constant daily incapacitating migraine headaches for 5 years. Seen by multiple headache clinics.

Key Physical Finding
48-year-old female. Neurological and musculoskeletal components within normal limits except for cervical hypertonicity, a various specific type of somatic dysfunction of the head, cervical, thoracic, lumbar, sacrum, and pelvis.

Diagnosis
Migraine cephalgia, tension cephalgia, somatic dysfunction of the head, cervical, thoracic, lumbar, sacrum, and pelvis.

Treatment Type
Osteopathic manipulation using indirect myofascial release, articulatory, and high velocity/low amplitude techniques and YNSA.

Frequency: Patient was seen over the next 2 years once a month and has been pain-free for 6 weeks at a time, with all treatments using cranial osteopathic manipulation, YNSA, and non-narcotic polypharmacology.

Details: Left Yin of YIN GB, LR, HT, PC, and KI. Right Yin of YIN HT, ST. Yin of YIN M-1.

Response
After initial cranial osteopathic manipulation, migraine pain diminished from 5/10 to 0/10 and tension headache pain diminished from 5/10 to 3/10. Post-YNSA, tension headache diminished from 3/10 to 0/10.

Leg Paresthesia

Chief Complaint
Low back pain and burning pain on the lateral aspect of the right leg that at times causes muscle spasm and pain in the lateral aspect of the right leg. The pain has been ongoing for several weeks.

History
Review of systems shows that the paresthesia is only noted in the lateral aspect of the right thigh and leg and does not extend to the foot. It covers more than one dermatone. MRI shows no herniated disc and is negative.

Key Physical Findings
Deep tendon reflexes were +2/+4, normal sensation to pinprick, coordination normal, normal gait. Somatic dysfunction was found with specific joint restrictions. L4 and L5 were rotated right sidebent left, with left sacral torsion present and a right anterior innominate. Left lower extremity has good muscle strength. Normal range of

motion. Right lower extremity has good muscle strength. Pain distribution that is consistent with the bladder channel. There is no dislocation, subluxation, laxity, or crepitation of any of the joints.

Diagnosis

Paresthesia, somatic dysfunction of the lumbar, sacrum, pelvis, and lower extremity.

Treatment Type

Osteopathic manipulation and YNSA acupuncture.

Frequency: One visit.

Details: Yang of YIN left GB and right GB; right D-1–6, D-leg.

Response

100% pain relief.

Lumbar Herniated Disk

Chief Complaint

Right hip and leg pain for the last 2 weeks. Celebrex 200 mg two twice a day. Pain in the leg not the hip, and leg is weak. Pain was 2/10.

History

48-year-old male with herniated nucleus pulposus L4–L5 by MRI 1 year prior.

Key Physical Findings

Deep tendon reflexes were +2/+4. Left quadriceps was 2/4 and right quadriceps was 0/4. Somatic dysfunction identified with left sphenobasilar synchondrosis torsion, C2 rotated left sidebent left, T4 rotated right sidebent left, L5 rotated right sidebent left, left sacral torsion, and anterior right innominate.

Diagnosis

Sciatica, old herniated disk (HNP) L4–L5 disc, somatic dysfunction of the head, cervical, thoracic, lumbar, sacrum, and pelvis.

Treatment Type

Osteopathic manipulative using indirect, myofascial release, muscle energy techniques, and YNSA.

Frequency: Weekly visits for 4 weeks.

Details: YNSA Yin right D-1–6.

Response

Resulted in 100% pain relief and remained symptom-free for 2 years.

Post-cerebrovascular Accident—Hemiplegia

Chief Complaint

Right-sided hemiparesis with contractions of the elbow, wrist, and fingers, decreased sensation of the lower extremities.

History

1.5 years ago experienced stroke causing left-sided weakness and lack of mobility during a cervical laminectomy with fusion.

Key Physical Findings

Several specific areas of somatic dysfunction were identified, including head, cervical, thoracic, lumbar, sacrum, and pelvis.

Diagnosis

Right hemiparesis and somatic dysfunction of the head, cervical, thoracic, lumbar, sacrum, and pelvis.

Treatment Type

Osteopathic manipulation using indirect, myofascial release and YNSA.

Frequency: Weekly.

Details: YNSA left Yin of YIN KI, BL and right Yin of YIN GB, BL, Yin of YIN M-1 left and right, M-2, M-3, right A, right C-1, and right Broca's aphasia point.

Response

Increased range of motion of the right upper and lower extremity immediately after placement of the needles.

Sciatica

Chief Complaint
Pain in the left leg radiating from the lumbar spine.

History
Onset several weeks prior. MRI shows L5–S1 bulging disc. Pain was 2/10.

Key Physical Findings
Deep tendon reflexes were +2/+4. Sensory is normal to pinprick. Positive Lasègue's sign. Somatic dysfunction was found with T2–T7 rotated left sidebent right, T8–T9 rotated right sidebent left, L2–L4 rotated right sidebent right, L5 rotated right sidebent left, left sacral torsion, right anterior innominate. Left and right lower extremity range of motion joint and muscle strength were within normal limits.

Diagnosis
Sciatica, bulging disc L5–S1, myositis, and somatic dysfunction of the thoracic, lumbar, sacrum, and pelvis.

Treatment Type
Osteopathic manipulation using indirect, high velocity/low amplitude techniques and YNSA.

Frequency: One visit.

Details: Yin of YIN left C-2.

Response
100% pain relief. Patient was instructed to resume normal activity. Patient was seen 1 month later with no recurrent sciatica or additional neuromusculoskeletal problems.

Sciatica with Reflex Sympathetic Dystrophy

Chief Complaint
Left sciatic pain of 5 months' duration.

History
50-year-old female with reflex sympathetic dystrophy (CRPS II) of the right foot. Spinal stenosis diagnosed by MRI of the lumbar spine.

Key Physical Findings
Review of systems was noncontributory. Areas of somatic dysfunction were found of the head, cervical, thoracic, lumbar, sacrum, and pelvis.

Diagnosis
Sciatica, spinal stenosis of the lumbar spine, RSD, and somatic dysfunction of the head, cervical, thoracic, lumbar, sacrum, and pelvis.

Treatment Type
Osteopathic manipulation using indirect, high velocity, low amplitude techniques and YNSA.

Frequency: Weekly for 8 weeks then monthly.

Details: Left Yin of YIN GB, KI, and right Yin of YIN GB, left Yin of YIN D-1–6, E, and right Yin of YIN D-1–6.

Response
After the fourth visit, patient had several days of 0/10 pain compared with the initial pain level of 8/10.

Tinnitus

Chief Complaint
Ringing in the ears for over 2 years and minimal hearing loss.

History
56-year-old female who had high-pitched ringing of the ears for the past 6 months.

Key Physical Findings

Noncontributory osteopathic structural examination found areas of somatic dysfunction of the head, cervical, thoracic, lumbar, sacrum, and pelvis.

Diagnosis

Tinnitus and somatic dysfunction of the head, cervical, thoracic, lumbar, sacrum, and pelvis.

Treatment Type

Osteopathic manipulation using indirect, myofascial release, articulatory techniques and YNSA.

Frequency: Follow-up visits show that the tinnitus stays away for hours to days.

Details: Left Yin of YIN GB, PC, and SI. Right and left tinnitus points.

Response

Immediate relief of tinnitus with each YNSA treatment, no permanent relief after 12 treatments.

Temporomandibular Joint/ Jaw Pain

Chief Complaint

Pain on both sides of jaw. Headaches. Pain was 3/10.

History

Jaw pain for 9 months after her wisdom teeth were pulled. She had difficulty opening her mouth.

Key Physical Findings

Opening 28 mm from incisor to incisor, crepitance of left and right TMJ. MRI shows anterior displacement of the disc.

Diagnosis

Temporal mandibular joint disease, myositis, somatic dysfunction of the head, cervical, thoracic, sacrum, pelvis.

Treatment Type

Osteopathic manipulation using indirect, myofascial release procedures and YNSA.

Frequency: Weekly for 4 weeks, then every other week for 4 weeks.

Details: YNSA Yin of YIN GB, PC, M-1, and TMJ point left and right.

Response

Resulted in improvement of opening to 34 mm. After six visits, opening increased to 40 mm. No pain after the fourth visit. MRI post-treatment shows the right condyle appears to be deformed, forward motion is restricted. No disturbance of TMJ disk is identified. Small joint effusion is visualized.

Whiplash

Chief Complaint

Complained of headache and neck pain particularly in the left side of the back of the head.

History

14-year-old gymnast landed flat on her back, hitting her head. Diagnosed with whiplash by her family physician.

Key Physical Findings

Diminished cranial rhythmic impulse, left sacral torsion, right lateral strain in the sphenobasilar synchondrosis, C2–4 rotated right sidebent right, T4–7 rotated right sidebent left, L5 rotated right sidebent left, right anterior innominate.

Diagnosis

Acceleration/deceleration injury/whiplash and somatic dysfunction of the head, cervical, thoracic, lumbar, sacrum, and pelvis.

Treatment Type

Osteopathic manipulation using indirect, myofascial release, high velocity, low amplitude, articulatory procedures and YNSA.

Frequency: Weekly.

Details: YNSA Yang of YIN GB, LR, HT, PC left.

Response

100% relief of pain post-treatment. Pain scale went from 6/10 pretreatment to 0/10 post-treatment. Maintenance treatment of four visits per year needed.

Poor Balance after Stroke

Chief Complaint

67-year-old female first seen in January with a chief complaint of weakness of the left side of the body with poor balance.

History

History of chief complaint is that of a prior stroke that occurred on September 2, and a second stroke that occurred in November of that same year resulting in left-sided hemiparesis and disequilibrium with minimal dysarthria.

Key Physical Findings

Active movement of the left forearm included supination 20 degrees, pronation 10 degrees, no wrist flexion or extension, no abduction or adduction, no finger or thumb movement. Shoulder movement allowed for flexion 10 degrees, abduction 10 degrees, adduction 10 degrees, and extension 0 degrees.

Other significant findings: acupuncture pulse was characterized as hollow and deep. Five Phase pulse diagnosis was (−1) HT, (=) SI, (+0.5) LR, GB, KI, and BL, (=) LU, LI, (+0.5) SP, ST, PC, and TB.

Diagnosis

The patient had many areas of somatic dysfunction of head, cervical, thoracic, lumbar, sacrum, and pelvis, with significant cranial restrictions.

Treatment Type

After cranial osteopathy was applied, YNSA neck diagnosis was positive for Yin of YANG, Brain, LR, PC, HT, GB, BL, SP, ST, and SI.

Frequency: Visits occurred twice weekly for 2 weeks and then weekly thereafter.

Details: YNSA treatment was: M-1 left and right, M-2 left and right, M-3 left and right, A-1–7 left and right, C-1 left and right, LR left and right, PC left and right, HT left and right, GB left; KI, BL, SP, ST, and SI right. All points taken in the Yin of YANG scalp position.

Response

Response after first treatment: upper extremity movement; supination improved to 30 degrees, flexion improved to 90 degrees, adduction was 90 degrees, abduction was 40 degrees

The next visit the patient had reported some improvement a few days after the last treatment, but recently unsteadiness has returned and the left hemiparesis continues.

YNSA diagnosis was Yin of YIN position and YNSA treatment consisted of M-1, M-2 left and right, M-3 left and right, A-1–7 left and right, B-1 left and right, C-1 left and right; in the Yin of YIN scalp position right, LR, PC, HT, GB, BL, SP, ST, SI, left PC, HT, GB, BL.

On third visit, hemiparesis had improved slightly, hand is showing some signs of discomfort, and the Yin of YIN scalp position was identified and Basic points M-1 left and right, M-2 left and right, M-3 left and right, A-1–7 left, C-1 left, E-1–12 left and right, D-1–6 right, Ypsilon point LR, PC, GB, KI, LU, all on the right and left PC, HT, KI, LU.

On the fourth visit, left arm is achy, hemiparesis persists, YNSA neck diagnosis showed Yin of YANG quadrant. Treatment in the Basic points was: M-1 left and right, M-2 and M-3, right LR, PC, GB, left LR, PC, HT, GB, KI, BL, TB, and LI.

On the fifth visit, left-sided weakness persists, but the range of motion had improved; flexion of the left upper extremity was 90 degrees, extension was 20 degrees, internal rotation 0 degrees, external rotation 0 degrees, abduction 90 degrees, adduction 20 degrees.

YNSA diagnosis was Yin of YIN quadrant and YNSA Ypsilon points on the right was GB, left LR, PC, GB, KI, BL, ST.

On the sixth visit (4 weeks of treatment), YNSA diagnosis was Yin of YIN, scalp points were taken of M-1 left and right, M-2,3, and A-1–7; right PC, HT, GB, KI, BL, TB, LI, ST, and LU; left PC, TB, GB, KI, BL.

On the seventh visit, flexion was 90 degrees, extension was 30 degrees, internal rotation was 15 degrees, external rotation was 5 degrees, abduction was 60 degrees, and adduction was 30 degrees.

YNSA found Yin of YIN scalp quadrant, Basic points were M-1 left and right, M-2,3, A-1–7, D-1–6; left B-1, C-1, right-hand Yin of YIN LR, PC, HT, SP; left was LR, PC, HT, GB, BL, and SP.

The eighth visit found range of motion slightly improved, overall with Yin of YIN on YNSA neck diagnosis, and Basic points needed were left A-1–7, left D-1–6, and E-1–12; left is LR, PC, HT, GB, and KI.

Results

With left hemiparesis as a result of two different strokes with the oldest being 4 months ago, significant range of motion improved in all of the cardinal ranges of motion of the shoulder. However, finger and hand dexterity did not change in the first six visits. Visits occurred twice weekly for 2 weeks and then weekly thereafter. The disease state can start in any one of the four quadrants, but the longer the disease is within the person's system, body, mind, and spirit, the higher it is in the yang area. Her condition started as Yin of YANG, then went to Yin of YIN, and in this case had a reversal back to Yin of YANG on one occasion, was treated and reversed to the ideal position for healing to occur in Yin of YIN.

Significance

YNSA is helpful in stroke rehabilitation and old, serious illnesses often progress from YANG to Yin of YIN.

Spinal Cord Injury

Chief Complaint

Pain in the lower abdominal area, burning and stabbing pain not related to abdominal disease after GI work up, pain was dermatomal L1–3.

History

A 24-year-old female, seen in February with T12 and spinal cord injury that occurred in January of the previous year due to a motor vehicle accident.

Key Physical Findings

Loss of sensation to pinprick in the lower abdomen T12 dermatome to sacrum. Loss of motor muscle control from T12 to sacrum, with resultant leg paraplegia.

Diagnosis

T12 spinal cord transaction secondary to trauma with resultant paraplegia of lower extremities.

Treatment Type

YNSA diagnosis was Yin of YIN condition with Basic points M-1 left and right, M-2,3, A-1–7, E-1–12, and right C-2; right LR, PC, GB, HT, BL, TB, LI, SP, ST; left PC, GB, KI, BL, TB, LI, SP.

Frequency: One visit per week for 3 weeks.

Details: Second visit: YNSA diagnosis was Yin of YIN, scalp treatment of the Basic points were: M-1 left and right, M-2,3, A-1–7, E-1–12, D-1–6, C-2; right LR, PC, HT, GB, LU; left LR, PC, HT, GB, KI, BL, and LU. Pain level was 0/10 after treatment.

Third visit: YNSA diagnosis was Yin of YIN, scalp treatment of Basic points left and right M-2,3, E-1–12, and C-1; no pain post-treatment.

Examination the following week noted that the pain had decreased. YNSA diagnosis was Yin of YIN, scalp treatment M-1 left and right, M-2,3, A-1; left LR, PC, GB, KI, BL, ST, SP; no pain post-treatment.

Response

Pain level diminished from a 5/10 to a 2/10 on the first visit.

Second visit was 1 week later, the patient reports improved feeling in her back and across the lower abdomen, pain level was 5/10, post treatment it was 0/10.

Third treatment 1 week later, the patient reported that the nerve pain had decreased, but was more prominent the night before, at the time of visit her pain level was 6/10, post treatment it was 0/10.

Significance

The paraplegia did not change since it was traumatic, severing of the spinal cord, but the lower abdominal pain abated after each YNSA treatment.

Neck Stiffness and Low Back Pain

Chief Complaint

A 63-year-old female seen in March with a chief complaint of neck stiffness, pain level is 2 on a 10 scale.

History

Past medical history includes cervical laminectomy with fusion C6–7.

Key Physical Findings

Positive YNSA neck diagnosis, somatic dysfunction, C1 rotated right, soft tissue changes of the lower cervical and upper thoracic region.

Diagnosis

Post C6–7 cervical fusion, 6 weeks, somatic dysfunction of the head, cervical, and thoracic.

Treatment Type

YNSA diagnosis was Yin of YIN, scalp Basic points utilized: M-1 left and right, M-2,3.

Frequency: Two visits.

Details: YNSA diagnosis was Yin of YIN with treatment of Basic points: M2, M3, A1-7 on the right; Ypsilon points on the right: LR, PC, GB, SP, ST, SI. A second visit was similar for the Basic points only.

Response

No pain post-YNSA treatment.

Four months later, she came in complaining of low back pain.

YNSA diagnosis was Yin of YIN, scalp treatment right D-1–6, left GB. Pain diminished from 2/10 to 0/10 with one treatment.

Significance

This is a good example of how often simple, acute flare-ups can be abated with only two or three YNSA needles.

Right Low Back Pain, Right Shoulder Pain

Chief Complaint

A 58-year-old female with a chief complaint of right low back pain, right-sided pain in the right shoulder of 3 weeks' duration.

History

The patient had a positive straight-leg-raising test on the right side.

Key Physical Findings

Areas of somatic dysfunction in the lumbar region of L4–5, along with left sacral torsion.

Diagnosis

The diagnosis of somatic dysfunction was made in that area along with sciatica.

Treatment Type

Osteopathic manipulative treatment was given using myofascial release, articulatory and high velocity/low amplitude techniques.

Frequency: One visit for YNSA.

Details: YNSA diagnosis was Yin of YIN, Basic points on the left and right at D-1–6, acupuncture Five Phase diagnosis had pulses with spleen pulse (–1.5), all other pulses (–0.5). Thus, she had a block between stomach (XI) and spleen (XII), acupuncture was given using ST-41, SP-1, and SP-9. The entry/exit points were used with SP-9 to technically transform a single Five Phase acupuncture treatment into a French Energetics treatment. YNSA D-1–6 Yin of YIN was used. This decreased the pain significantly.

Response

The patient returned 2 weeks later complaining of low back pain. Somatic dysfunction was found at L4–5 on the right and osteopathic manipulation was used to relieve this problem, the pulse diagnosis was normal. YNSA diagnosis was normal.

Significance

This shows the integration between various styles of acupuncture as well as how YNSA can be used as an adjunct to other modalities, whether it be manual techniques, French Energetics acupuncture, or Five Phase acupuncture.

Migraine Headaches

Chief Complaint

A 53-year-old-female with a chief complaint of common migraine headaches, head tremors, and pill-rolling tremors.

History

Five years prior, dizziness occurred after an inner ear infection, tinnitus resulted in the right ear and tremor of the left hand began. Neck and shoulder pain started two years prior to first visit.

Key Physical Findings

Positive YNSA neck diagnosis, somatic dysfunction of the head, cervical, thoracic, lumbar, and sacrum, the right temporal was locked in internal rotation, the left temporal was held in internal rotation, right sphenobasilar synchondrosis torsion.

Diagnosis

The diagnosis is Parkinson's along with common migraine. Meningioma of the right cranial nerve VIII, acoustic.

Treatment Type

YNSA every two weeks. Migraines improved after second visit.

Frequency: Every two weeks.

Details: YNSA findings were Yin of YIN, scalp points Basic on the left and right M-2,3, on the left HT, GB; and on the right GB.

Response

Migraine pain abated but pill-rolling tremor remained.

Significance

Parkinson's disease is a disease that needs comprehensive treatment not just YNSA. Common migraine patients have received immediate relief with just one YNSA treatment and multiple treatments for chronic conditions.

Ankle Numbness, Hip Discomfort

Chief Complaint

A 52-year-old female with a chief complaint of numbness/tingling in the left ankle, right hip discomfort, and a history of left knee pain and left patella tracking dysfunction.

History:

Left ankle sprain two weeks prior.

Key Physical Findings

The osteopathic diagnosis was internal rotation strain of the ankle and somatic dysfunction of the lower extremity. Neurological examination found deep tendon reflexes +2/+4 with no abnormalities to pinprick of the ankle. Coordination of the ankle, heel, knee, and shin was normal.

Diagnosis

The diagnosis was sprain/strain with neuritis of the left ankle.

Treatment Type

Osteopathic manipulative treatment was given along with YNSA.

Frequency: One visit.

Details: YNSA diagnosis was Yin of YIN, left GB, PC.

Response

YNSA treatment resulted in no pain.

Significance

This simple sensory symptomatic case shows that Basic points are not necessarily always required, if the Ypsilon points achieve the result. The GB and PC are energetically paired structures, the GB courses through the ankle, and the GB channel controls the muscles and tendons, thus, this case shows the congruity of TCM, French Energetics, and YNSA.

未濟 ䷿ 未濟 ***Wèi jì***

Not Yet Fulfilled—Fire Above, Water Below

"Not Yet fulfilled.
There is prosperity and smoothness,
For the yielding attains the central place.
Little fox, almost across the river.
It is not yet past the central line.
Wets its tail. Nothing is favorable.
There is no continuation at the end.
Although all lines are not in their proper place,
Yet the strong and the weak still respond to each other."[2]

References

1. Huang A. The Numerology of the I Ching: A Sourcebook of Symbols, Structures, and Traditional Wisdom. Rochester, VT: Inner Traditions; 2000: 86
2. Huang A. The Complete I Ching. Rochester, VT: Inner Traditions; 1998: 494–495

Appendix

YNSA Basic Points, Ypsilon Points, and Neck Diagnostic Charts

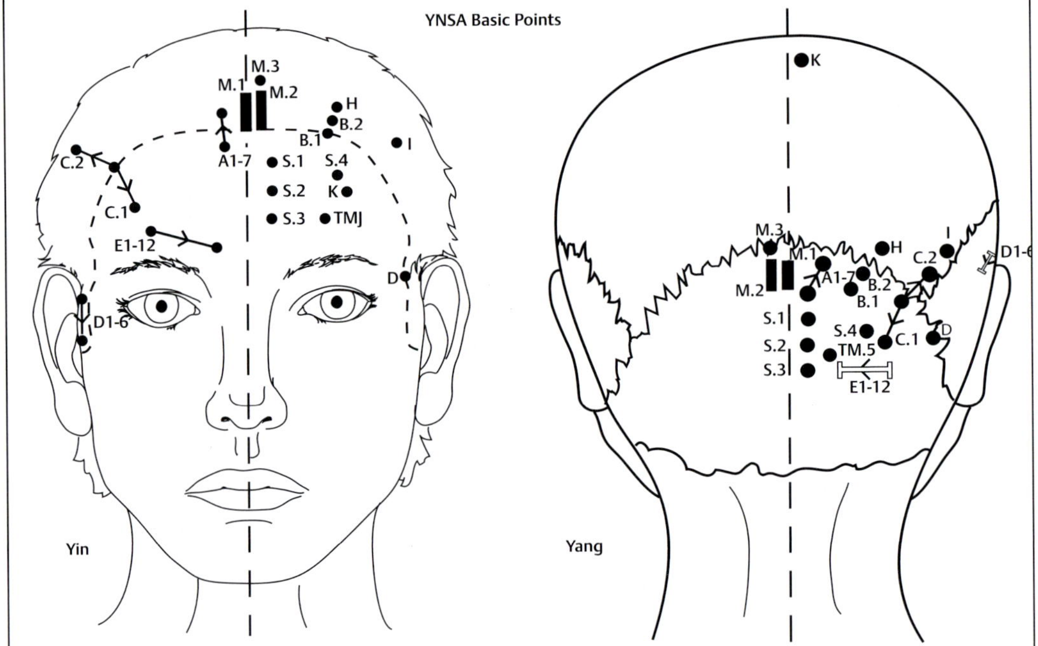

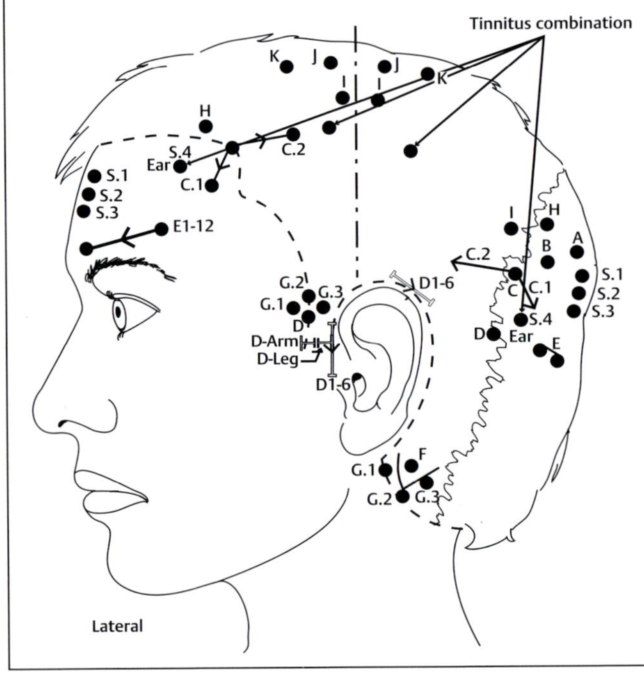

A1-7	Cervical spine; C 1–7
B.1	Shoulder
B.2	Foot paresthesia
C.1	Forehead, shoulder, upper arm, elbow, forearm, wrist, fingers
C.2	Scalp, hip, leg & knee
D1-6	Lumbar spine; L 1–5 + sacrum
D	Low back
E1-12	Thoracic spine; T 1–12 chest
F	Sciatica
G.1	Knee; lateral
G.2	Knee; medial
G.3	Knee; proximal
G	Knee
H	Lumbar, extra point
I	Lumbar, extra point
J	Feet, dorsal
K	Lumbar, HNP
M.1	Basal ganglia
M.2	Cerebellum
M.3	Cerebrum
S.1	Eye
S.2	Nose
S.3	Mouth
S.4	Ear
TMJ	Temporomandibular joint

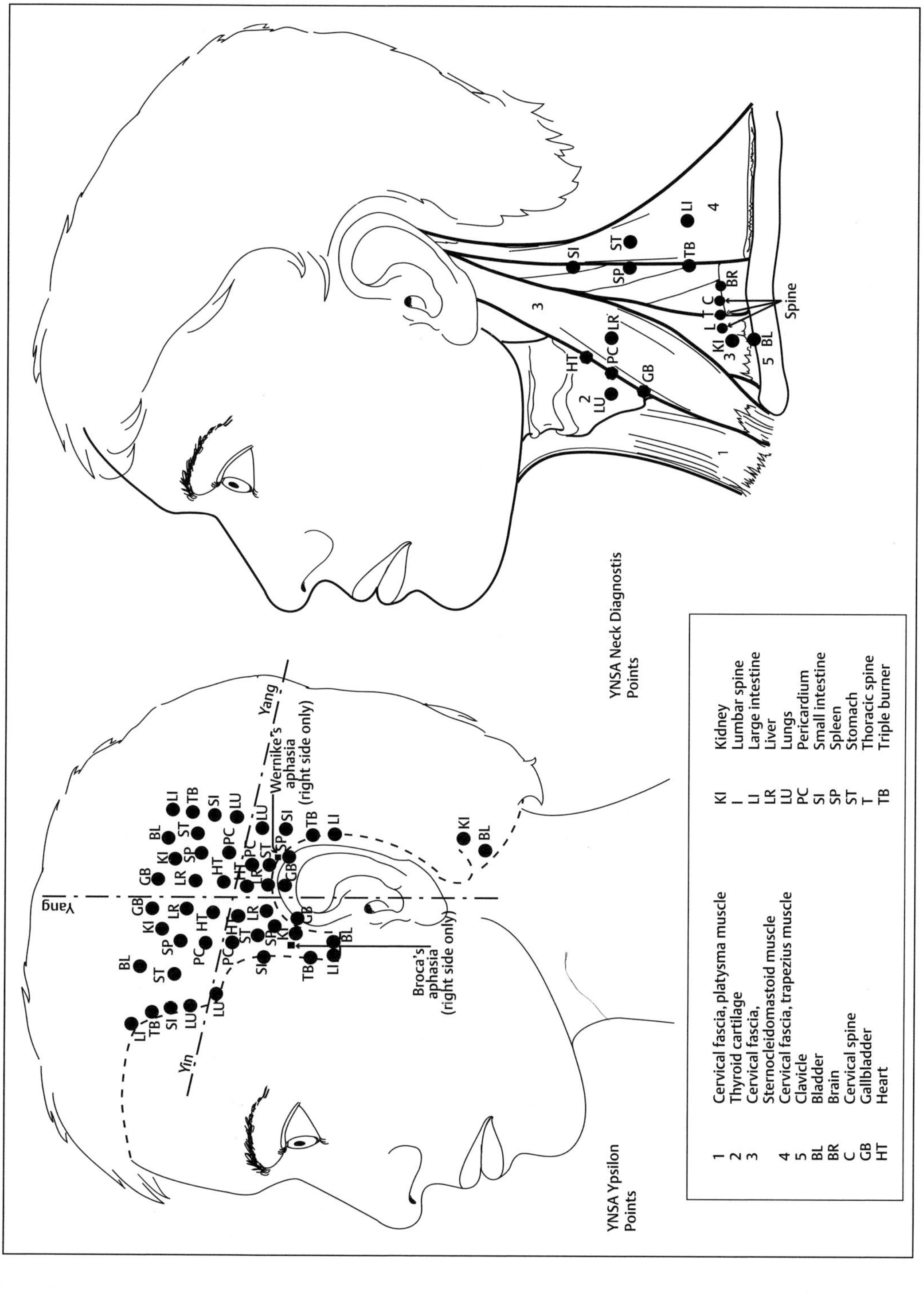
YNSA Ypsilon Points
Yang
Yin
Wernike's aphasia (right side only)
Broca's aphasia (right side only)
YNSA Neck Diagnostis Points
Spine
1 Cervical fascia, platysma muscle
2 Thyroid cartilage
3 Cervical fascia, Sternocleidomastoid muscle
4 Cervical fascia, trapezius muscle
5 Clavicle
BL Bladder
BR Brain
C Cervical spine
GB Gallbladder
HT Heart
KI Kidney
L Lumbar spine
LI Large intestine
LR Liver
LU Lungs
PC Pericardium
SI Small intestine
SP Spleen
ST Stomach
T Thoracic spine
TB Triple burner

YNSA Musculoskeletal Progress Note

Page ____

YNSA Acupuncture/Musculoskeletal Progress Note

Date________ **Name**________________________________ **ALLERGY: NKADF**________________

MEDS:________________

S: Chief Complaint

Location______________________ Duration______________________ Quality______________________

Severity: Pain_____/10_____________ Context______________________ Modifying Factors______________________

O: Review of Systems: check mark=normal X=abnormal circled items below are positive findings

__ General / Constitutional __ Abdomen / gut __ Eyes / head __ Genital ________________

__ ENT __ Blood / lymph / immune __ Skin / breast __ Neurologic ________________

__ Heart / vascular __ Mental Health __ Chest / Lung __ Endocrine ________________

__ Musculoskeletal __ All Other Negative see problem list reviewed__________

Past Medical, Family, Social History / ADL: *no changes since last visit*________________

***BP**_____/_____sit/supine **Pulse**_______reg/irreg **Resp**_______/min **Temp**_____**Wt**_____**Ht**_____**Age**__________

***General Appearance:** Well Nourished, *normal*, obesity, overweight, unkempt________________

***Cardiovascular:** *Yes/No* Edema____________Varicosities______________Temp______________Pulses__________

***Lympadenopathy:** *None*, neck, axillae, groin________________

***Gait and Station:** *Normal*, antalgic, ataxic, festinating, high steppage, hysterical, scissor, toppling, spastic,

Limp L/R______________Listing L/R____________ cane, crutches, walker, wheelchair, neonate/toddler

***Mental Status:** Oriented: *time, place, person*, Mood: happy, *normal*, depressed, anxious, agitated, angry____________

***Neurologic:** Left: DTR; biceps /4, triceps /4, Quad /4, Achilles /4, Babinski +/-, SLR: +/- sitting, +/- supine

Right: DTR; biceps /4, triceps /4, Quad /4, Achilles /4, Babinski +/-, SLR: +/- sitting, +/- supine

***Sensation:** *normal* to pin, hyper/hypo to pin ________________

***Coordination:** *normal* / abnormal: finger to nose, heel / knee / shin, rapid alt. movements arm/legs, fine motor: *left / right*

***Chinese Pulse:**

LEFT		RIGHT	
SI	HT	LU	LI
GB	LR	SP	ST
BL	KI	PC	TB

Reviewed with patient: Lab, EMG-NCV, X-ray, MRI, CT report / films

See in Chart: History, Physical, Structural and Acupuncture examination forms

Head & Neck:

A. Muscle Strength: /5 *good*, weak, hypertonicity, hypotonicity, atrophy________________

B. OMM: impaired or altered joint motion *WNL*________________

Head:________________

Cervical:________________

C. ROM *WNL* Flex_______Ext_______L lat rot______R lat rot______L rot______R rot______Pain *Yes / No*

D. Joints *Yes/No* discoloration, subluxation, laxity, crepetation ________________

***Skin:** *normal*, rashes, lesions, café-au-lait spots, ulcers, scar, tattoo________________

Spine, Ribs, Pelvis:

A. Muscle Strength: /5 *good*, weak, hypertonicity, hypotonicity, atrophy________________

B. OMM: impaired or altered joint motion *WNL*________________

Thoracic:________________

Lumbar:________________Ribs:__________

Sacrum:________________

Pelvis:________________

C. ROM *WNL* Thoracic/Lumbar: Flex____Ext____L lat rot____R lat rot____L rot____R rot____Pain *Yes / No*

D. Joints *Yes/No* discoloration, subluxation, laxity, crepetation ________________

***Skin** *normal*, rashes, lesions, café-au-lait spots, ulcer, scar, tattoo________________

Page _____

Left Upper Extremity

A. Muscle Strength: /5 *good*, weak, hypertonicity, hypotonicity, atrophy________
B. OMM: impaired or altered joint motion *WNL*________
C. ROM: *WNL* Flex____Ext____Int rot____Ext rot____ABd____ADd____Pain *Yes / No*
D. Joints: *Yes/No* discoloration, subluxation, laxity, crepetation ________
***Skin:** *normal*, rashes, lesions, café-au-lait spots, ulcers, scar, tattoo________

Right Upper Extremity

A. Muscle Strength: /5 *good*, weak, hypertonicity, hypotonicity, atrophy________
B. OMM: impaired or altered joint motion *WNL*________
C. ROM: *WNL* Flex____Ext____Int rot____Ext rot____ABd____ADd____Pain *Yes / No*
D. Joints: *Yes/No* discoloration, subluxation, laxity, crepetation ________
***Skin:** *normal*, rashes, lesions, café-au-lait spots, ulcers, scar, tattoo________

Left Lower Extremity

A. Muscle Strength: /5 *good*, weak, hypertonicity, hypotonicity, atrophy________
B. OMM: impaired or altered joint motion *WNL*________
C. ROM: *WNL* Flex____Ext____Int rot____Ext rot____ABd____ADd____Pain *Yes / No*
D. Joints: *Yes/No* discoloration, subluxation, laxity, crepetation ________
***Skin:** *normal*, rashes, lesions, café-au-lait spots, ulcers, scar, tattoo________

Right Lower Extremity

A. Muscle Strength: /5 *good*, weak, hypertonicity, hypotonicity, atrophy________
B. OMM: impaired or altered joint motion *WNL*________
C. ROM: *WNL* Flex____Ext____Int rot____Ext rot____ABd____ADd____Pain *Yes / No*
D. Joints: *Yes/No* discoloration, subluxation, laxity, crepetation ________
***Skin:** *normal*, rashes, lesions, café-au-lait spots, ulcers, scar, tattoo________

A: Assessment; ________

____

____

____

P: Plan; 1. ***Yes / No*** **Yamamoto New Scalp Acupuncture** ***Yin / Yang of YIN / YANG*** **Scalp / Chest / Pubis**

Basic Points: MI *Left / Right* M2 M3 A1-7 B1 B2 C1 C2 D D1-6 E1-12 F G1 G2 G3 H I J K P S1 S2 S3 S4 Tinnitis Aphasia TMJ Z-5

Ypsilon Points:
Left LR PC HT GB KI BL TB LI SP ST SI LU
Right LR PC HT GB KI BL TB LI SP ST SI LU

2. ***Yes / No*** **Acupuncture**; Chinese________

____

3.________

____

____

____

____

Response to treatment; PAIN____/10________
Return to Office: ____**Day(s)** ____**Week(s)** ____**Month(s) PRN Discharge Dr.**________

Internet Resources

Acubriefs

Acubriefs is sponsored by the Medical Acupuncture Research Foundation (MARF). Its purpose is to make the most comprehensive database of references on acupuncture in the English language available online.

http://www.acubriefs.com

Acupuncture.com

Something for everyone. A great site with consumer, student-level, and practitioner-level information.

http://www.acupuncture.com

Acupuncture for Arthritis

http://nccam.nih.gov

American Academy of Medical Acupuncture

An organization open to medical doctors who practice acupuncture. This site also has general information, books, and tapes for the public.

http://www.medicalacupuncture.org

Auriculotherapy Certification Institute

ACI is North America's only organization offering certification specifically in auriculotherapy, auricular acupuncture, and auricular medicine.

http://www.auriculotherapy.net/

Auriculotherapy Network

Information on the work of Dr. Paul Nogier of France.

http://www.nogier.info

DrFeely.com

Links for practitioners to various health-related topics treated with acupuncture.

http://www.drfeely.com

The National Acupuncture Detoxification Association

The National Acupuncture Detoxification Association is a nonprofit association that conducts training and provides public education about the use of acupuncture as an adjunctive treatment for addictions and mental disorders.

http://www.acudetox.com

National College of Natural Medicine

National College of Natural Medicine is the oldest accredited naturopathic medical college in North America.

http://www.ncnm.edu

NIH Consensus Statements

Contents discuss the efficacy of acupuncture, its role in combination with other interventions, its biological effects, how acupuncture can be appropriately incorporated into the health system, and future directions for research.

http://consensus.nih.gov/1997/1997Acupuncture107html.htm

Oregon College of Oriental Medicine

Oregon College of Oriental Medicine trains master's and doctoral students, conducts research, and treats patients at clinics on campus and in the community.

http://www.ncnm.edu

Pacific College of Oriental Medicine

The largest TCM college in the United States with campuses in San Diego, Chicago, and New York, Pacific offers master's degrees in Traditional Oriental Medicine.

http://www.pacificcollege.edu/

"The Meridian System and the Mechanism of Acupuncture"

This scientific article by Charles Shang, Boston University School of Medicine, presents a theoretical model of how acupuncture might work.

http://www.vxm.com/21R.65.html

Yamamoto New Scalp Acupuncture (YNSA)

Yamamoto New Scalp Acupuncture is a fast and easy-to-learn method, among other applications, for the treatment of acute strokes and represents a valuable complement to conventional schemes of treatment.

http://www.ynsa.com/English_version/english_version.html

Index

Page numbers in *italics* refer to illustrations or tables

A

B

C

Y

Z